WORKING WOMAN'S BEAUTY BOOK

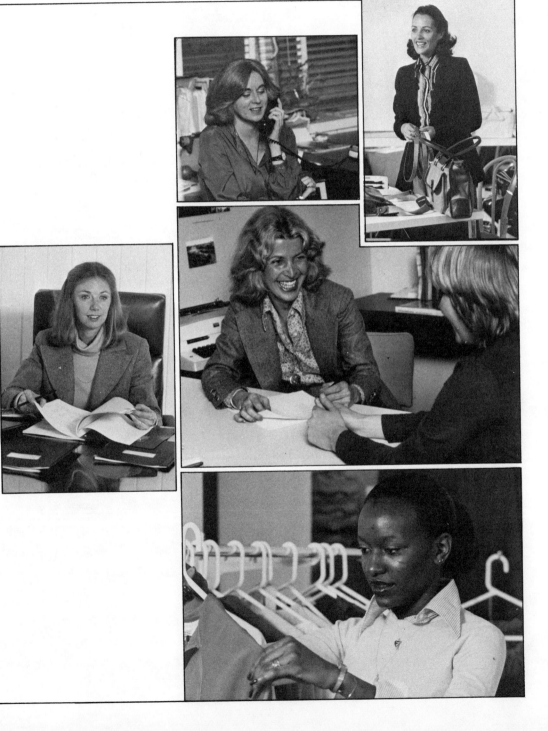

THE **HELENA RUBINSTEIN** LIBRARY OF BEAUTY

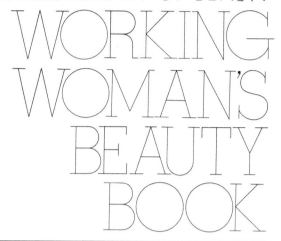

WORKING WOMAN'S BEAUTY BOOK

Sharron Hannon

𝔰𝔻 STEIN AND DAY/*Publishers*/New York

First published in 1979
Copyright © 1979 by Helena Rubinstein, Inc.
All rights reserved
Printed in the United States of America
Stein and Day/*Publishers*/Scarborough House
Briarcliff Manor, N.Y. 10510

*Library of Congress Cataloging
in Publication Data*

Hannon, Sharron.
    Working woman's beauty book.

        1. Beauty, Personal.   2. Women—
Health and hygiene.
3. Women—Employment.   I. Title.
RA778.H35   646.7   78-19959
ISBN 0-8128-2517-9

Photographs: Steve Weiner

Drawings: Paula Joseph

Design: Michaelis/Carpelis Design Associates

To this working woman's best friends:
a husband and a mother who
help and support in countless ways

The Helena Rubinstein Library of Beauty
Series editor: Barbara Bonn

Working Woman's Beauty Book
Sharron Hannon

Beauty Makeover Guide
Judith Ross and Susan Acton

Prime of Life Beauty Book
John Foreman
with the Helena Rubinstein Beauty Experts

CONTENTS

Working
Woman's
Beauty
Book

WORKING WOMAN'S BEAUTY BOOK

Introduction

More than 41 million women work outside the home today—a stagger-
ing increase of 17 million over the number of working women in 1960.
Not only are more women in the work force than ever before, but they
are moving into occupations formerly closed to them and beginning to
think in terms of choosing a career rather than just taking a job. Women
now see work as a continuous, integral part of their lives, not just a
temporary situation to be abandoned when marriage and babies come
along.

This flood of women into the work force has been called the "single
most outstanding phenomenon of our century" by economist Eli
Ginzberg, and there is no doubt that the phenomenon is shaking up the
business world. What used to be a men's club is being slowly but
relentlessly integrated by females. Men who have been relating only on
a social level suddenly find they have to learn to deal with women on a
professional basis as well. It's not an entirely comfortable adjustment
for either sex, but, as usual, the burden of easing the situation seems to
be falling primarily on women. Women are the ones being counseled on
how to dress and how to act in order to be taken seriously by male'
bosses and co-workers.

In the past year or so, several books and innumerable magazine
articles have addressed themselves to the question of what women
should wear to work if we want to make it past the typing pool and
toward the boardroom. While these writings went to great lengths to
lay down precise principles of acceptable attire (plain pumps, yes;
open-toed shoes, no), there were invariably two shortcomings. One, the
advice was too limited and too dull (must we really confine ourselves to

drab business "uniforms" just when men are acquiring much more freedom in their attire?). Two, the focus on clothing was often so single-minded that it ignored the woman inside the clothes.

We decided that clothes do not make the woman—at least, not entirely. The face, the hair, the hands, the body, the overall state of health and fitness are also of great importance. To exclude any of these from consideration is to risk ruining the total picture.

And so, *The Working Woman's Beauty Book*. This comprehensive guide is dedicated to taking care of *all* of you, based on the premise that you don't have to deny the fact that you are female in order to be successful. We'd like to believe that women can be bright and ambitious *and* attractive. Note that we're not talking about prettiness here, but a way of putting yourself together so you always look your best from head to toe.

Self-styled "wardrobe engineer" John Molloy, one of those who contend that in order to be serious you must dress seriously, advises women to avoid makeup, except perhaps lipstick, on the job. We take issue. While the principle of looking natural is certainly a good one to follow, Mr. Molloy, being a man, does not understand one basic beauty truth of contemporary American society: It takes more makeup to look like you're wearing less. Cheryl Tiegs, who epitomizes the natural look of the seventies, carries around a makeup case with at least 25 items essential to her.

We're not saying that every woman needs to go to these lengths, but it is important to understand which products are right for your skin type and coloring and how to use them. To prove that a beauty routine may be simple, we selected six working women, each with a different type of job and a different life style. We sat them down with Helena

Rubinstein makeup expert Suzanne Quinn and gave each a tailor-made beauty plan to fit her special needs. All were delighted with the results. Part I of this book deals with the specifics of these sessions, while Part II provides loads of general advice for you to pick and choose from.

Our two main considerations in offering suggestions to working women are (a) time and (b) money. We recognize that any woman putting in a full day's work and trying to maintain a meaningful personal life doesn't have a lot of time to devote to complicated beauty routines. But what many women perceive to be a problem of time is actually one of *technique*. Once you master some basic skills and practice them frequently, you'll find that beauty routines can be accomplished in a matter of minutes.

We're also aware that the average working woman is not a princess with limitless funds to spend on herself or a staff of servants to take care of home and children while she tends to personal pampering. We've tried to suggest when it might be a good idea for you to pay for professional beauty services and when you can do it yourself. We do feel that the way you look is an important investment for a working woman, because it indicates how you see yourself and your career. If you decide to spend a week's salary on a smashing outfit to wear to the office, you can certainly afford to spend a fraction of that on a good makeup or skin-care product that will enhance the way you'll look in that outfit.

We are concerned about your inner workings, too. And this book has plenty of suggestions on how to eat right, select an exercise program, relieve stress, and get a good night's sleep. We feel that keeping fit is crucial to looking good and feeling good and that, in the end, good health is a working woman's most important beauty asset.

PART ONE

**The Working
Woman's
Beauty
Problems**

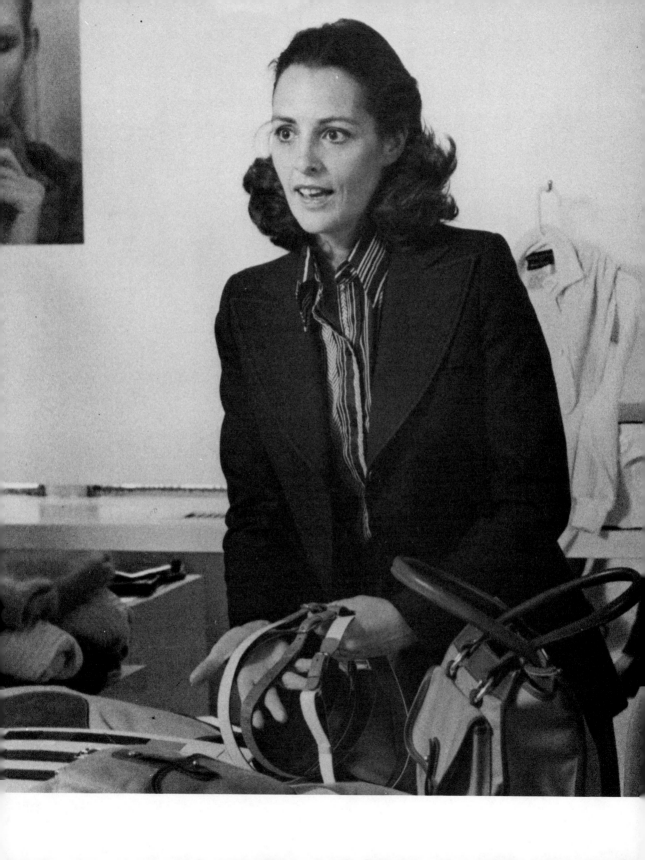

CHAPTER ONE

Finding Time for Yourself with Kids and a Career

SUBJECT: LINDA HODGSON, VICE PRESIDENT, MARKETING

By the time Linda Hodgson gets to her office in the morning, she already needs a rest. "I have to have my coffee and a few moments of peace and quiet before anything else happens," she says. "Otherwise I'd fall apart." No wonder. By 9 A.M. Linda has already put in a hectic two-and-a-half hours getting herself and her husband and two children ready to start their days.

"The hours before 8:30 are terrible, especially since my family are all big breakfast eaters," she says. "I have to do everything the exact same way each morning or I can't get it all done. If the slightest thing happens to mess up my schedule, like getting a phone call, the whole day is thrown off."

Linda's alarm goes off at 6:30. She staggers out of bed and down to the kitchen to pour orange juice or section grapefruit. Then she dresses quickly, sets her hair with electric rollers, and does her makeup. "I suppose I could save some time if I had shorter hair that was easier to take care of," says Linda. "But I like this style, so I make the extra effort." The next step is to get the children up. While she dresses two-year-old Lindsay, Bucky, five, climbs into his clothes with exhortations for speed from his mother.

Then it's time to wake husband Marley, who is, according to Linda, "absolutely no help in the morning. I don't know what happened to women's lib at our house, but it obviously ignores us until after 9 A.M."

With the kids started on their fruit or juice, Linda gets into the serious business of making breakfast, which at the Hodgsons' includes eggs, bacon, cereal, toast, and rolls, and for Marley, instant breakfast on top of everything else. While all this is being gobbled up, Linda makes Bucky's lunch and tosses laundry into the washing machine.

At 8:30 she rushes out the door to take Bucky to school just as the housekeeper rushes in. "Of course, this whole process is complicated in winter, when I have to get boots, coat, hat, scarf, and mittens on Bucky," Linda adds.

After a morning like this, office work can indeed seem relaxing. Linda runs the Manhattan sales office of a leather goods company that manufactures men's and women's accessories: belts, attachés, bags, umbrellas, and wallets. Linda likes to wear classic clothes to work: blazers, silk blouses, and skirts belted with the company's latest design. She is particularly enthusiastic about the belts and other products since they happen to be designed by her husband.

The company was a dream of the Hodgsons' back in the late 1960s, when the couple was living in the Midwest and Linda was handling public relations for a major Chicago bank. In 1970 they moved to New York to launch the business. As usual with such ventures, the first few years were lean ones, but Linda kept things afloat with another job in banking. In November 1972, with the family business beginning to do well, Linda took time out to have her first child. But she was back to work by January, this time as part of the family business. She continued working throughout her second pregnancy, taking just eight weeks off when the baby was born.

"Theoretically, I'm now working four days a week, but it rarely turns out that way," says Linda. "I usually have to come in to the office for at least a few hours on the fifth day. Then, too, my hours are supposed to be 9 to 5, but it's usually closer to 5:45 when I leave. I do like to be home by 6 or 6:30 at the latest, so I can give the kids dinner. I want to make sure they know I'm Mommy."

Among Linda's office duties are planning marketing strategy along with her husband, working on advertising and public relations, preparing the company's catalogue and sales brochures, handling special customer problems, and supervising the New York sales office and a staff of four. Marley comes in to the sales office once or twice a week, but spends most of his time at the company factory overseeing plant operations and managing the business. "If we were in the same place with the same responsibilities, we might have problems working together," says Linda. "But with Marley running the factory and me running the office, it works out very well."

One of Linda's current projects is designing a tag to put on leather and twill bags and luggage to detail the quality production methods used in making each item. "With lots of products today, packaging is everything. The product itself actually costs very little to make. With us, it's just the opposite. Our products are very expensive. The fine

"I have to do everything the exact same way each day or I can't get it all done."

leathers and other materials and the workmanship that goes into our leather goods are most important and that's where the money goes. For instance, all the solid brass hardware for the belts, bags and luggage that Marley designs are made at a foundry in Milan, Italy, that works exclusively with us."

Although initially a men's accessories company, the Hodgson's began moving into the women's field two years ago. Their belts, handbags, attachés, and umbrellas have attracted the attention of *Vogue* and *Glamour* magazines. Most recently the company entered the boys' market with a line of belts. The men's, women's, and boys' goods are sold all around the country, usually to fine specialty shops but also to some department stores like Bloomingdale's and Neiman Marcus.

To ensure that their lives are not all work and no play, the Hodgsons have a regularly scheduled night out each week. (The babysitter comes every Wednesday evening, rain or shine.) They go to dinner and the movies or pick up last-minute theater tickets. For additional recreation, Linda recently joined a tennis club and plays once a week. "The nice thing about the place is that they'll set up matches for you," says Linda. "All I have to do is call up a day ahead of time and tell them when I'd like to play. Before or after the match, I take a half-hour tennis lesson. I'm a low intermediate aspiring to play better. I just wish I could play more often, especially since, other than walking to work occasionally, this is the only exercise I get."

And, of course, those morning workouts.

●

Linda arrived at Helena Rubinstein headquarters feeling less than gorgeous, having just come from the dentist's office, where she'd had 18 stitches removed from her mouth following oral surgery a few days before. "Help! I look awful!" she pleaded.

Linda has naturally good looks—including high cheekbones and clear skin with refined, tight pores—so helping her wasn't tough at all. Training director Suzanne Quinn began by removing Linda's makeup with cleanser. Then she applied a moisturizer in a clear shade. Since Linda's skin tone is basically balanced, there was no need to use a color-corrective one.

The next step was to use an eye oil wrinkle stick, a solid lubricant in a lipstick-size case, to dot under Linda's eyes and in the light creases between her nose and the corners of her mouth. Though her skin type is normal, these are two dry areas that need special attention. The oil stick helps to soften them as well as lubricate.

Suzanne applied liquid foundation in warm tawny to give Linda's skin a finer finish and chose a rosy shade of cream blush for cheek color. Another good shade when Linda wants to wear dramatic colors would be a bright cherry red. To go with earth tones, Suzanne suggested bronze cheek color. Whatever the shade used, blusher should be applied high on the cheekbones and winged up and out toward the hairline.

Before making up Linda's eyes, Suzanne used concealer in a medium shade in the under-eye area. Linda was astounded by the results. "I've always had dark circles under my eyes that I couldn't do anything about," she said. "Whenever I've used a cover-up it always came out looking like chalk." Suzanne explained that it is important to use concealer in a tone to match your skin. Dark circles under the eyes are hereditary, so there is nothing that can be done to make them go away. But they can be successfully camouflaged by tapping the concealer lightly to blend it in.

Suzanne also recommended that Linda not use any foundation or moisturizer in the eye area. Using moisturizer under the eyes before bedtime is one of the causes of "puffy eyes" the next morning, she said. The eye oil and concealer combination is all that is necessary under the eyes, while the lid and brow area do best with just a shadow base—a cream applied beneath shadow to keep the color true and lasting.

Because Linda has large, pretty eyes, Suzanne wanted to play them up by using three shades of shadow instead of the two she recommends for most women. She stroked a light gray on the lid area, a darker gray in the crease, and sheer white on the brow bone for a highlighter. Next she used a smoky eyeliner near the base of the upper lashes to make them look thicker. Suzanne does not like to use liner at the lower lashes, because she thinks this tends to close up the eyes rather than make them look bigger. She did, however, apply mascara to Linda's upper and lower lashes. For the upper lashes, she uses one stroke down and then one stroke up. For lower lashes, the mascara wand is held vertically, and color is applied to one lash at a time.

For everyday skin care, Suzanne recommended that Linda use cream cleanser or a gentle cleansing bar, a toner, and a moisturizer day and night. She also suggested a creamy clay mask once a week to help tighten and brighten the skin and keep it in its best condition. Eyelash, eye and neck creams used on a nightly basis, provide extra TLC and should be staples on everyone's list.

By the end of the session, Linda was glowing, inside and out. "I feel like a new person," she said. "Do you think you could come by my house about 6:45 A.M. and do this for me every day?"

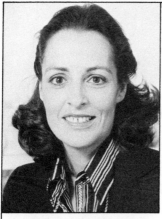

LINDA HODGSON
Age: 36
Eyes: Brown
Hair: Brunette

Skin Type: Normal
Recommended Skin Care:
   Cleansing: cream cleanser or mild soap
     eye makeup remover
   Toning: toner
   Day Care: moisturizer
     eye oil wrinkle stick
   Night Care: lightweight cream
     eyelash cream
     eye cream
     neck cream
   Special care: facial mask

Skin Tone: Medium complexion with a
basically balanced tone
Recommended Makeup:
   Foundation: warm tawny
   Cheek Color: rose, cherry red or bronze
   Concealer: medium
   Lip Color: rose, cherry red or bronze
   Lid Color: light gray
   Pressed Powder Eyeshadow: dark
    gray/sheer white
   Eyeliner: charcoal gray
   Lash Color: black
   Shadow Base

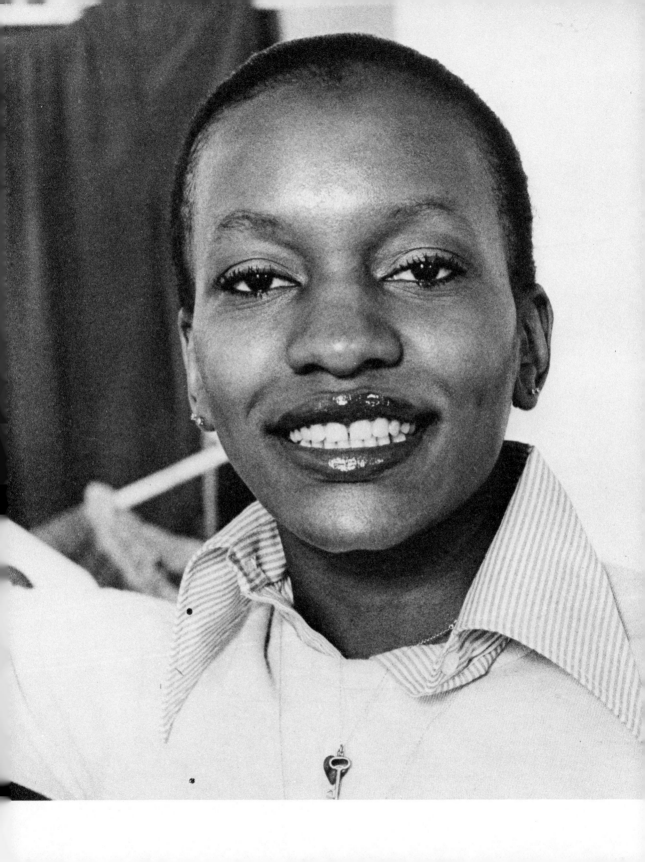

CHAPTER TWO

Creating a
Professional Image

SUBJECT: GRACE KELLEY, FASHION BUYER

Grace Kelley has little more in common with her famous namesake than good cheekbones. But she is perfectly satisfied with being who she is: 20 years old, single, and launching a career that she's excited about. Just four-and-a-half weeks and 15 interviews after graduation from a fashion professional school, Grace landed a job as an assistant buyer for a company in New York City's garment district.

"It's my first real job," she says. "Actually, I'm only a junior assistant buyer right now. But I hope to move up fast. I'm learning all about the business by writing up orders for stores, doing the follow-ups, like finding out why something wasn't shipped on time, and handling cancellations."

While most of her morning is spent on the phone and doing paperwork, there is plenty of action in the afternoon. At about 1:30 P.M. every day, Grace is sent out "into the market"—the teeming fashion center located on Manhattan's West Side—to drop off orders to as many as 30 different manufacturers. Her rounds must be completed by a 5 P.M. deadline, when she returns to the office to write up confirmations.

"Sometimes I get tired psychologically before going into the market," says Grace. "But once I'm out there, I feel fine. Somehow I get energized. One of the things I love about the job is getting to see the different styles as they come in. We're buying clothes six months before they'll appear in the stores. I'm a trendy dresser, so I like being ahead of things."

In the business she's in, Grace can get away with wearing the latest Seventh Avenue looks to the office, but when she was searching for a job she thought it best to tone down her personal style. "I tried to be conservative," she says. "I wore a suit with a skirt to all my interviews. The placement office at the school I attended sponsored seminars on how to dress and how to present yourself when you were job hunting. I always went to them and I'm glad I did. Of course, at my first interview I was so nervous. But after a couple of them, I felt like a pro. Handling questions came easier each time.

"My major was fashion merchandising, but I went on interviews for several different positions, some clerical, some involving part-time modeling. I was caught off guard once when I was applying for a clerical position and the interviewer asked, 'But what do you really want to do?' At first I was afraid that if I told him my real ambition, he'd think I wasn't interested in the job he was offering—and I always wanted to come across as wanting the job I was interviewing for. But I decided that if I was honest, he would see that my objectives were good and that I had potential. So I said, 'I want to be a buyer.' I still think it was the best thing to do.

"Another tricky situation in the interviews was when I'd be asked questions about my personal life—if I had plans to get married and so forth. Of course, it wasn't usually put just like that, but I knew what they were driving at. I'd say, 'Gee, I'd better check with the placement office to see if we're supposed to give out that kind of information.' The interviewer would usually drop the topic."

Grace believes herself to be the type of woman who will not let marriage interfere with her working life. While she dreams of being a wife and mother someday, that vision is coupled with being a career woman.

"I think I can do it," she says. "My mother did. Right now she's working as the head nurse at a V.A. hospital and earning her master's degree as well. She's behind me in my career plans 100 percent. She's proud of me, and I'm proud of her. She set a good example and taught me to be self-sufficient."

Grace apparently has the courage of her convictions, having already turned down two marriage proposals. "Maybe in a year or a year and a half I might be ready to start thinking about getting married, but right now my main objective is to get my career started and booming."

Grace shares the same apartment she lived in when she was in school with her old roommate. "I lived in a dorm when I first came to school, but after a semester I moved out and got a place of my own." Her typical weekday begins at 6 A.M., when she rolls out of bed for 20 minutes of "slimnastics"—sit-ups, leg lifts, deep breathing, and so forth. Then she makes her bed and takes a shower. She allots 15 minutes for cleaning and treating her face, another 15 minutes for applying makeup. Her hair is quickly done by pulling it into a knot at the back of her neck. Then she gets into her clothes, which are always laid out the night before.

Breakfast is a quickie, a handful of vitamins with juice or milk, and Grace is off to work. She likes to arrive at 8:30, though her day doesn't

"Right now
my main objective
is to get my
career started
and booming."

begin until 9, in order to have some time to get organized. There are 12 people in her office, a merchandising manager, three buyers, and their assistants, and the desks are "all crammed together" in one large room.

Grace rarely takes time for lunch, preferring to grab a frozen yogurt from a fast-food stand as she dashes around making her afternoon rounds. If she has one bad habit in the way she takes care of herself, this is it. Breakfast and lunch should be much more substantial. She would be wise to choose some of the fast, low-calorie food selections described in Chapters 8 and 10. She admits that she has the typical single working girl's attitude of not wanting to bother much with food. The half-size refrigerator in her apartment is always understocked, and, as she says, "The only time I really eat well is when I go out to dinner or to visit my relatives in Queens." Poor nutrition can take its toll on a person's health and good looks, and Grace agreed it was time to change some of her eating habits. She certainly walks and exercises enough not to have to worry about gaining weight.

In addition to her daily workouts at home and on the job, Grace takes an occasional dance class. She studied ballet for six years when she was growing up and was in the modern dance club at school. "Sometimes, even now, when I get home from work I just turn on the stereo and dance."

The very first thing Grace does when she gets home is to take off all her makeup. "Then I have something to eat and read the newspaper," she says. "In the evenings I go out or rap with my roommate or just relax with a good book or new magazine. On work nights I go to bed early—9 P.M. sometimes and certainly no later than 11. If I didn't, I'd be too tired to get up the next day."

In her sleeping habits, as in the rest of her life, Grace is always thinking ahead.

●

Grace's biggest beauty problem, one shared by many black women, is excessively oily skin. Not only does the oiliness make her face shine as the day goes along, but it occasionally causes acne flare-ups. She's tried combatting the condition during the day by powdering her face every couple of hours, but Suzanne Quinn had some other ideas. Rather than treating a skin problem with a makeup product, she suggested that Grace try a treatment product—something that would actually help, not just cover up the problem. If she carries around a small plastic bottle filled with astringent and some cotton pads, she has, in effect, a traveling treatment kit that she can use to help cool and freshen her face and tighten pores. All she has to do is saturate the cotton and rub it over her forehead, nose, and chin a couple of times a day. She should also carry face blotters, small squares of linen which can be purchased in drug stores, to soak up extra oil without disturbing her makeup.

If Grace wants to wear foundation, she should choose a water-based formula. But, since her skin tone is fairly even, she doesn't really need the coverage. Suzanne felt that Grace should concentrate on emphasizing her cheekbones and her eyes. She chose cognac blusher to use on Grace's cheeks and up around her forehead. The color was applied high on her cheekbones and blended out to the hairline and up to the temples.

For Grace's eyes, Suzanne began by dotting eye oil wrinkle stick on the under-eye area, a spot that needs lubrication even for oily skin types. She then used a deep-toned concealer to even out dark circles there. She applied creme base on the lid and under the brow to help keep shadow colors true all day. A golden walnut lid color was stroked on Grace's lid, then a smoky brown was used in the crease for contouring.

Because Grace has large lids, she can easily use two or three shadow colors. Suzanne advised that she choose earth tones when wearing neutral colors, plum tones to go with blues and mauves. She recommended a smoky plum and frosted peach as an eye-color combination that would go with a rosy cheek color. To keep cheek color lasting as long as her eye color, Grace can apply cream blush and then top it with a dusting of powdered blush.

For a finishing touch to the eyes, mahogany eyeliner was applied at the base of both upper and lower lashes. Though Suzanne generally finds that using liner under the eyes closes them up too much, Grace's are large enough to handle the look. Black mascara was then used to enhance her already thick and curly lashes. Suzanne also suggested that Grace pluck some stray hairs from her brow and even the line with a pencil.

Grace can wear a deep rich burgundy, a browned red, or a wine color on her lips. A gloss slicked over the color enhances their fullness. If Grace wants them to appear less full, she can use a pencil to outline just inside the natural lip line, and then fill in with color.

Suzanne's suggestions to Grace about skin care included washing her face at least twice daily with a cleansing bar formulated for oily skin or with a water activated face wash. Cleansing should be followed with an application of astringent and this by a touch of moisturizer to dry areas. When black skin becomes too dry it takes on an ashen look; skin cells turn lighter in color as they dry out. Affected areas should be moisturized twice daily. Suzanne did not recommend blotting lotion, a special formula that provides oil control while protecting vital moisture. Though ordinarily a good product for oily skin, she felt it might look chalky on Grace. To control excess oil and unclog pores, she recommended using a clarifying mineral mask, an astringent clay-type mask, at least three times a week.

When Grace is troubled by acne flare-ups, she was cautioned to keep her hands off her face. Her skin tends to scar easily from poking, resulting in a host of tiny black spots. She was told not to use strong acne medications containing resorcinol, since these will also cause the spots.

The marks are, of course, only temporary and fade with time. Suzanne advised that Grace not put any makeup over them, as this would only emphasize the condition. She suggested a gentle facial bleach, which is formulated not only to lighten dark spots, but to safely fade uneven pigmentation of face, hands, and body.

By paying a little more attention to her special skin care needs, this Grace Kelley can be just as stunning as a princess.

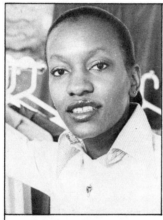

GRACE KELLEY
Age: 20
Eyes: Brown
Hair: Black

Skin Type: Oily
Recommended Skin Care:
   Cleansing: soap for oily skin
     or water activated face wash
     eye makeup remover
   Toning: astringent
   Day Care: moisturizer
     eye oil wrinkle stick
   Night Care: eyelash cream
     eye cream
     neck cream
   Special Care: astringent facial mask
     facial bleach

Skin Tone: Deep complexion with a
          basically balanced tone
Recommended Makeup:
   Cheek Color: cognac or rose
   Concealer: deep
   Lip Color: burgundy,
        browned red or wine
   Lid Color: golden walnut and
        smoky brown
        smoky plum and peach frost
   Eyeliner: mahogany
   Lash Color: black
   Shadow Base

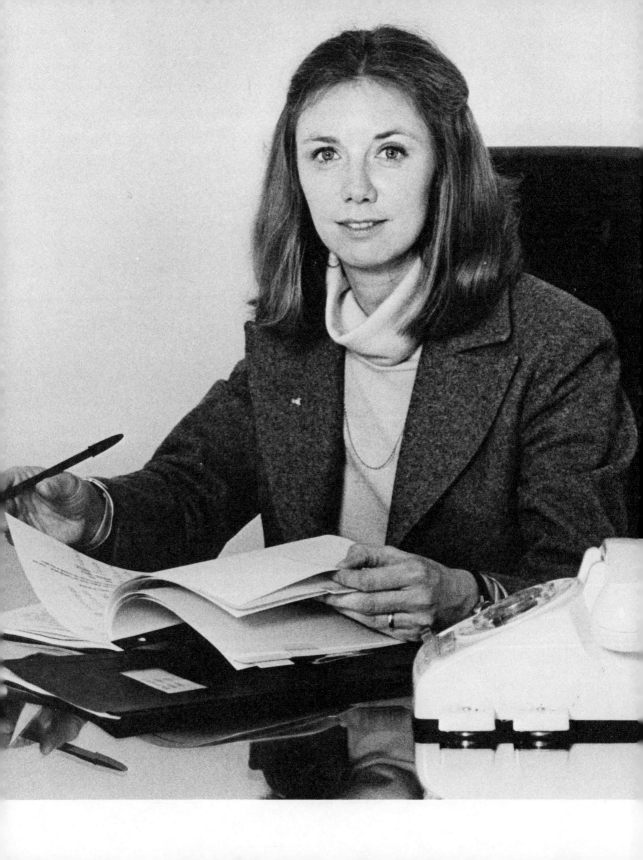

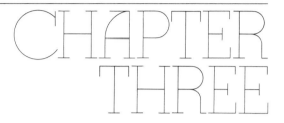

Handling Business Travel with Style

SUBJECT: SUSAN FOWLER, BANK EXECUTIVE

Susan Fowler considers herself "an aggressive person," but sees this as a distinctly constructive quality. She believes her aggressiveness is not only responsible for her rapid climb up the corporate ladder of the large metropolitan bank where she works, but credits it with helping her land her new husband.

"Gus and I lived in the same apartment building," she says, "and we happened to be riding the elevator together one evening. I decided I was going to say something to him first, so when he pushed the button for the 14th floor, I asked him how the view was from up there. I explained that my apartment was on a lower floor and looked out on the back of another building. We chatted for a couple of moments, then I had to get out.

"The next morning, he was on my elevator again, and this time he struck up the conversation. We ended up walking to the subway and then riding to work together."

These days Susan and Gus always ride to work together, but on a commuter train from their new suburban home instead of on the subway. "When we decided to get married, we also decided that we would buy a house. We started looking and figured that as soon as we found one we liked, we'd plan the wedding. We wanted to find a house in A-1 condition, since both of us are too busy with our jobs to be able to put time into fixing up a place. We were lucky to find one that was perfect. The people who owned it before us had just finished painting it, inside and out. We didn't even have to do any cleaning."

The only drawback was that there was only one bathroom. "We do have to coordinate our use of the mirror in the morning," says Susan. Usually she is the first one up, and she finds that it takes her exactly 30 minutes to get dressed, do a quick makeup routine, brush out her shoulder-length straight hair, and grab some toast and coffee. She likes to take a train that gets her to the office by 8:15 A.M. so she has a leisurely half hour to drink another cup of coffee and read the *Wall Street Journal* before she begins her paperwork.

"I have never been a 9-to-5 person," she says. "I always get in earlier and leave later. I think the amount of time you're willing to put in on a job has to do with your interest in it. Obviously I'm interested in mine."

Obviously, too, her interest has been noticed—and rewarded. Since joining the bank after graduation from college in 1970, Susan has moved rapidly through the ranks, from personnel to credit training to international banking to her new position in the metropolitan division. At age 29, she has reached the level of assistant vice-president, a noteworthy accomplishment in an industry where only two percent of the senior jobs are held by women.

Susan credits some of her progress with being in the right place at the right time. "I was the first woman hired for the bank's management training program in the personnel division. They gave me a special project of revising and rewriting the personnel policy manual. It was supposed to take three to six months. But when I got into it, I discovered that the manual hadn't been reviewed in 25 years. A lot of the policies were very outdated and needed changing rather than rewriting. I ended up working on it for 13 months. It was a real chore, but I learned a lot and got to meet people from all over the bank."

That project completed, Susan was assigned temporarily to the training department to help devise a program for clerical supervisors, and from there moved into recruiting. "I went into recruiting on a test basis in December of 1971," she says. "I was the first full-time female recruiter the bank had. Luckily for me, the recruiting manager never treated me as someone to be protected. My travel schedule was as difficult as the next guy's, and I was expected to handle all kinds of interviews, even of older men and M.B.A.s. I had to be extremely professional and know exactly what I was doing. Still, some people held my age and the fact that I was a woman against me. I was 24 at the time, and I remember one 30-year-old Vietnam veteran who refused to be interviewed by me."

Despite such occasional problems, Susan persevered, and in October of 1972 was made director of the bank's recruiting staff, a position she held for two years.

"I did so much traveling when I was a recruiter that I was hardly ever home. I'd just have time to dump out one suitcase of dirty clothes and repack with clean ones. I remember times when I wasn't able to catch a plane and ended up taking a train or driving all night to get to my next morning's appointment. But it was a really good experience. I certainly

"I did so much traveling, I'd just have time to dump out one suitcase of dirty clothes and repack with clean ones."

learned to take care of myself."

All of Susan's travel experience came in handy when she was transferred to the international division and assigned along with a group of other officers to handle accounts in Southeast Asian countries. She made her first trip overseas—to Hong Kong, Malaysia, and Thailand—in October 1976.

"I was gone five weeks and only took one suitcase," she recalls. "When I travel I wear the same sort of clothes I do in the office, but since I only pack a few changes, everything must be carefully coordinated. You can't afford to take clothes you'll wear only once or twice. I brought along mostly suits. The climate was warm in the countries I visited, but there was a lot of air conditioning. With suits, I could simply slip the jacket on or off to adjust to the temperature. For dinner, I brought jersey print dresses. They can go anywhere, and they take up almost no room in a suitcase.

"When I'm on a long flight I wear slacks on the plane to be more comfortable. And I sit in first class whenever the trip takes more than seven hours. From Tokyo to New York nonstop is 14."

Despite her globe-hopping schedule, Susan managed to be home long enough to get married last summer. Then in January she asked to be switched to the bank's metropolitan division. The decision hinged upon both personal and professional considerations.

"If I had stayed in international, I would have been asked to take an overseas position. And though Gus probably could have arranged to come with me, I still would have been traveling about 75 percent of the time from my overseas base. Then, too, I was interested in the metropolitan division because there is a lot of personal responsibility and authority involved."

So for now, Susan has her feet happily planted under her desk. Though she doesn't rule out the possibility of some domestic or international jaunts on behalf of her present corporate clients, she hopes to spend most of her time at home, sweet home.

●

Susan's combination skin type is shared by many women. Her cheeks are dry, while the area around her nose is slightly oily. With her blonde hair and blue eyes, her skin tone is fair and she needs some color to keep from looking pale and washed out. But like many blondes, she was reluctant to venture out of the pastel color range, fearing that more vivid shades would overpower her. Suzanne Quinn set out to change her mind.

Starting with suggestions for day-to-day skin care, Suzanne advised cleansing with a water activated face wash, a cleanser that is rinsed off rather than tissued off. This should be followed by two applications of toner, one to remove the last traces of cleanser and the other to tone and brighten the skin. An astringent facial mask, used twice a week, should take care of any excess oiliness and unclog and refine pores, too.

Because Susan's skin tone is basically balanced, she doesn't need any color corrective to even it out. Suzanne chose moisturizer in a natural shade to use as a base for a warm bisque foundation. When Susan is having a special problem with oiliness, as in the summer or when traveling, she might also use blotting lotion under her foundation to keep it shine free.

Like many women, Susan was also making the mistake of using moisturizer around her eye area. Suzanne explained that the water in moisturizers is absorbed into the skin and causes puffiness. She switched Susan to an eye oil wrinkle stick, a lubricant that stays on the surface of the skin. A fair-toned concealer was used over the eye oil stick and patted in to blend.

For Susan's cheek color, Suzanne chose a vibrant, pinkish shade, blending it carefully so the color looked natural. For lips, a rosy transparent shade was used. When Susan first saw the lip color, she protested it was too dark. She was happy to find, however, that the color stroked on very sheer and was far more flattering to her than the white-based lipstick she had been wearing. She was surprised again when Suzanne did her eyes. After applying shadow base, she chose gray for the lids instead of the blue Susan was used to wearing. She explained that gray provides a contrast to Susan's blue eyes, making their color stand out more. In addition, a neutral shadow color is generally more flattering for a daytime look. Charcoal gray liner was used at the base of Susan's upper lashes, but not of the lower lashes. Instead, a bit of shadow was smudged in the outer corner of the lower lashes. Suzanne then used a light coat of black mascara on Susan's upper lashes and on the outside corner of her lower lashes.

For a finishing touch, translucent powder in a fair shade was dusted lightly all over Susan's face to give her skin a refined finish and help keep her makeup fresh throughout the day.

When Susan goes straight from work to a business dinner, she can redo her makeup using more dramatic colors for evening—more vivid cheek and lip colors, darker eye shadow shades. Suzanne encouraged her to experiment to find the best look that would play up her fair skin. By becoming as aggressive with color as she is with other aspects of her life, there's no chance that Susan will ever go unnoticed.

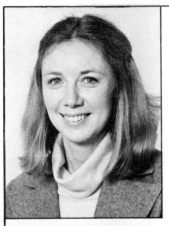

SUSAN FOWLER

Age: 29
Eyes: Blue
Hair: Blonde

Skin Type: Partly dry, partly oily
Recommended Skin Care:
   Cleansing: water activated face wash
     eye makeup remover
   Toning: toner
   Day Care: moisturizer
     eye oil wrinkle stick
   Night Care: moisturizer
     eyelash cream
     eye cream
     neck cream
Special Care: astringent facial mask

Skin Tone: Light complexion
   with a basically balanced tone
Recommended Makeup:
   Foundation; warm bisque
   Cheek Color: vibrant pink
   Concealer: fair
   Loose Face Powder: fair
   Lip Color: transparent rose
   Lid Color: dusky charcoal
   Eyeliner: charcoal gray
   Lash Color: black
   Shadow Base

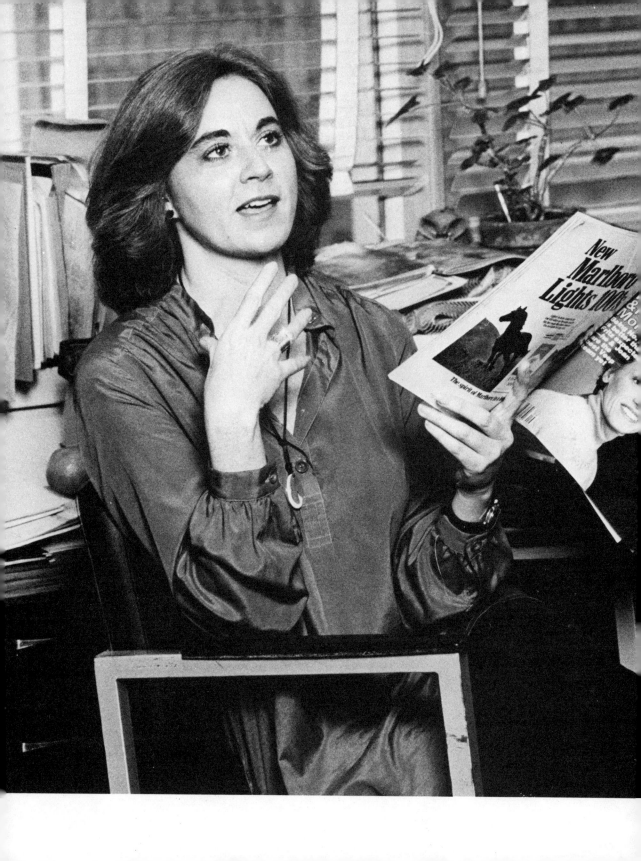

CHAPTER FOUR

Looking Fresh When You're on the Go All Day

SUBJECT: ALEXANDRA MEZEY, MAGAZINE RESEARCHER

Sandy Mezey has just spent $30 on a pair of running shoes. With her schedule, she should probably wear them round the clock. Among the activities that keep her hopping: a part-time job, master's degree studies, and a freelance career as a writer/photographer.

Her work week begins with two 12-hour-plus days as a researcher on the staff of a national magazine. Mondays and Tuesdays she works from 10 A.M. to around midnight, though quitting time is not always predictable. She is sometimes stuck at the office till 2 or 3 A.M. trying to close a difficult story.

"I have to check the accuracy of everything the writer says in an article," Sandy explains. "It involves reading background material, sending a lot of wires to verify facts, and making a lot of phone calls."

On Mondays, Sandy uses her dinner break to trot across town to a literature course that is part of her studies toward an advanced degree.

"The program is called Master of Arts in Liberal Studies," she says.

Working
Woman's
Beauty
Book

"Rather than training in a specialized field, the MALS program offers interdisciplinary courses of study, everything from art and literature to economics. At the New School for Social Research, where I study, the program is structured around the history of ideas. It is really exciting to me. My undergraduate degree was pretty much limited to education, so I feel this degree is rounding me out.

"Taking the course during working hours is pretty strange sometimes. One evening I was working on a story that involved trying to find out if Evel Knievel really hit someone with a baseball bat. Then I went to class and we discussed Plato and what makes a civilized man."

Sandy finds that working such long shifts can take its toll. She likes to dress comfortably, preferring pants and loose tunic shirts to more tailored skirts or dresses. Her naturally thick hair is worn parted simply down the center. "I start the day pretty well put together, but look progressively worse as the hours go by. I try to reapply my lipstick and blusher because having some bright color on my face makes me feel better. But sometimes I look in the mirror and get so discouraged I think, 'Why bother?'

"I'm usually wrecked from 4 to 9 P.M. Then I start feeling better, maybe because eating dinner picks me up. Of course, having the class on Monday is a good break. When I finally leave the office at night I always feel grimy, and I take a shower when I get home, no matter what time it is."

Wednesday is Sandy's day to take it easy. She sleeps late, then strolls over to a neighborhood pâtisserie for tea and croissants. "I sit and read the paper and feel among the leisured."

Looking fresh
when you're on
the go all day

Such moments are short-lived, however, for there is usually studying to do before her Thursday evening literature class. "The master's program I'm working on usually takes three years, but I'm hoping to do it in two by going to summer school. Since I've been working for the same company for 10 years, I have six weeks' vacation coming, and that's how I'll use it. I'm hoping to go to another campus for summer school, so I can get out of the city environment for awhile."

Sandy plans to write her final paper for the program on some aspect of photography, a subject near and dear to her heart. Her own picture taking, combined with her writing skills, has helped supplement her income from time to time. She has sold three freelance articles, accompanied by her photos, to major magazines. "All three stories came out of vacation trips I took—to a tennis camp in Massachusetts, down the Colorado River in a raft, and on a group bike trip through Vermont."

She is currently preparing another essay on her latest adventure, a trip to Ireland with her mother and two sisters. "It was a *Roots*-type journey for us, since my mother is Irish. We visited relatives in Kenmare and saw the graves of my great-grandparents. The best part for me was that my mother and sisters and I were alone together for the first time since we'd grown up. Their husbands stayed home to take care of the children."

Sandy's photography is not limited to illustrating her travel stories. She took a series of portraits at an old age home for an independent study course, and, she also shot her niece's ballet recital. "At Christmas I gave her Jill Krementz's book, *A Very Young Dancer,* which she loved. Then after her recital, I put her photos, which I printed myself, into a

"I start the day pretty well put together, but look progressively worse as the hours go by."

Looking fresh
when you're on
the go all day

similar book all about her."

Sandy's passion for picture taking also led her to another part-time job. On Thursdays she spends a couple of hours before lit class at a photography magazine putting together lists of exhibits. "It's a volunteer thing, but I feel I get something out of it. It keeps me in touch with what is going on in photography. I meet a lot of nice people and get invitations to shows and openings."

With all the running around town that Sandy does, you wouldn't think she's need any more. But she thinks so. "I've just started jogging a half hour in the morning three days a week," she says. "I used to swim at the Y regularly, and I enjoyed that. I even competed in the Master's Swim Program and won some medals. But the chlorine was drying out my hair, and I decided I was ready for a change of pace. Of course, I'll also be playing a lot of tennis in the summer."

Does Sandy ever do anything for pure relaxation? "Oh, yes. I practice TM intermittently. Sometimes I meditate at work in a conference room or the ladies' room, but it's hard to settle down to it. Maybe I'll try going on a meditation weekend sometime."

The question is, can she slow down long enough?

●

"I'm not much of a makeup person," Sandy told Suzanne Quinn before the start of her session at Helena Rubinstein. "I never wear foundation, and I only started wearing eye makeup recently. Of course, I did get pretty good results with that. A lot of people commented on it.

"What I am concerned about is my skin. It seems to be getting 'bloppy.' That's the only word I can think of to describe it. I've been putting on more moisturizer, and I even started doing some chin exercises. I guess I've started feeling conscious of my age, that I'm closing in on 40."

Suzanne outlined a basic skin-care routine to suit Sandy's partly dry, partly oily skin. It starts with using either a water activated face wash or mild soap in the morning and at night. Both are low-alkaline and won't strip the acid mantle from the face. Sandy was advised to follow this cleansing by using a toner all over her face. Though some combination skin types need to use an astringent in the oily T zone (the forehead, nose, and chin area), Suzanne felt this would be too harsh for Sandy. A toner stimulates and freshens skin without stripping it.

The next step was to apply blotting lotion to keep Sandy's skin looking fresh and shine free. The blotting lotion was applied to the oily areas of Sandy's face, lightweight emulsion to the dry areas. Because her skin has a tendency toward sallowness, both products were chosen in a warm color-corrective tone.

The final skin-care touch was to apply eye oil wrinkle stick in the under-eye area. Because there is no natural elasticity in the skin there, it was dabbed on very gently.

At night, Sandy can follow pretty much the same routine, except that after cleansing and toning she should apply just moisturizer rather than the blotting lotion. Suzanne also suggested that Sandy massage in neck cream nightly, beginning at the throat and working up to the chin with

Looking fresh
when you're on
the go all day

long strokes. The neck and throat area is poor in oil glands, and this treatment will help keep it supple.

Since Sandy doesn't like foundation, Suzanne eliminated that step but had some other advice for a natural daytime look. She suggested Sandy use a cream or powder blush high on her cheekbones, extending it up toward the temples. She also recommended that Sandy dust over her moisturizer with a bit of translucent powder to give her skin a more refined look and to serve as added protection from the environment. She showed Sandy how to tap a makeup brush against her wrist to shake off excess powder so that she gets the lightest covering possible.

Suzanne dotted concealer under Sandy's eyes to cover the circles there, then used shadow base on the lid area. She chose a shadowy pink for Sandy's lid and a plum shade for the crease above it. She extended the darker shadow out a little past the outside corner of the eye and then brought it in, to make Sandy's eyes look larger.

Though Sandy had been using eyeliner, Suzanne felt that this closed up her eyes and made them look smaller. Instead, she decided to play up Sandy's thick, curly lashes with several thin coats of mascara. She stroked a brown shade both under and over the upper lashes, but used it only in the outside corner of the lower lashes—again to open up the eyes as much as possible. A bit of lip gloss finished off Sandy's new "no makeup" look.

Because of Sandy's long working hours, Suzanne suggested that she might look and feel better if she repeated a shortened version of her morning skin-care routine sometime during the late afternoon. She

could wash her face without disturbing her eye makeup, then reapply
toner, moisturizer, cheek and lip color.

"I guess that might revive me from my usual 4 P.M. slump," said
Sandy. "Do you suppose it would help beat the bloppies, too?"

Looking fresh
when you're on
the go all day

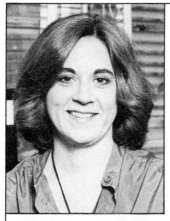

ALEXANDRA MEZEY
Age: 38
Eyes: Brown
Hair: Auburn

Skin Type: Partly dry, partly oily
Recommended Skin Care:
    Cleansing: water activated face wash
      or mild soap
      eye makeup remover
    Toning: toner
    Day Care: blotting lotion (warm shade)
      moisturizer (warm shade)
      eye oil wrinkle stick
    Night Care: moisturizer
      eyelash cream
      eye cream
      neck cream
    Special Care: astringent facial mask

Skin Tone: Light to medium complexion
    with a basically cool tone
Recommended Makeup:
    Cheek Color: peach
    Loose Face Powder: translucent
    Concealer: medium
    Lip Color: plum
    Pressed Powder Eyeshadow:
      plum/shadowy pink
    Lash Color: brown
    Shadow Base

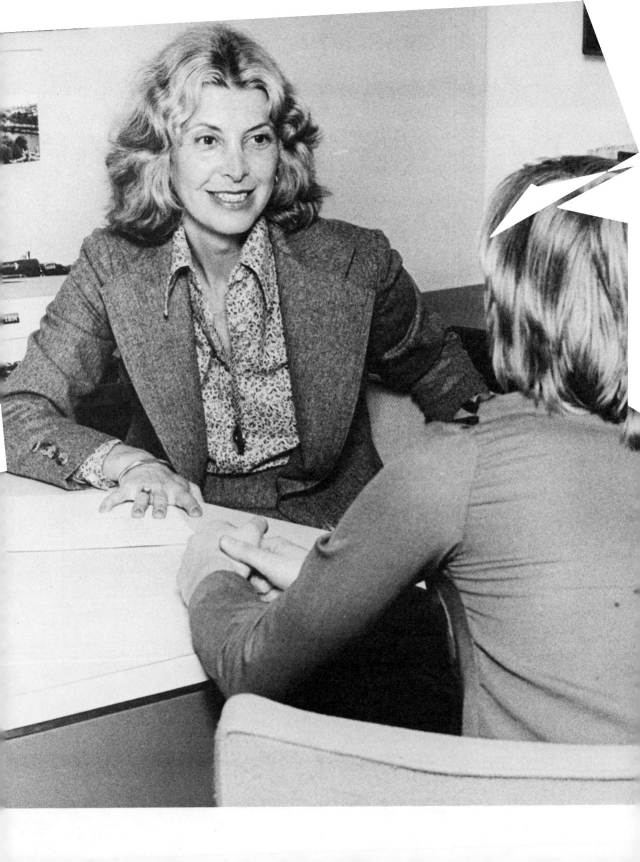

CHAPTER FIVE

Making the Switch from Housewife to Jobholder

SUBJECT: KIM DREZNER, COLLEGE RECRUITER

Kim Drezner, 42-year-old mother of four, went looking for a job last year. It was, she makes clear, a move prompted by necessity rather than choice.

"I wasn't going back to work seeking 'self-fulfillment' or because I felt I had to prove something," says Kim. "It was strictly a matter of survival. Divorced women don't get enough child support. I had to make some money."

Like many women surveying the job market after years spent raising children, Kim found the outlook bleak. "It seemed like every job I looked at was either incredibly dull, paid too little money, or demanded too much time. I still wanted my kids to be my number-one priority, so that limited the hours I was willing to put in on any job. Commuting was definitely out."

Still, in the beginning, Kim did trek into the city to make the rounds of employment agencies. "It was just awful," she says. "The prerequisite for any job seemed to be speed typing. Everyplace I went they immediately sat me down in front of an electric typewriter to take a typing test. I'd get completely flustered and end up with all the keys jammed. Meanwhile, all the other applicants would be whizzing through an entire page.

"I guess it was silly, but I was determined to get a job on my own. I didn't want to ask any of my friends to pull strings for me. Of course, now I know better, and if there is a next time, I'll make use of all the connections I have."

After several months of fruitless searching, Kim was sitting in her kitchen one Thursday doing a newspaper crossword and feeling discouraged. Then she noticed a small ad just above the puzzle: COLLEGE ADMISSIONS OFFICER WANTED. The school was a small one located in another state, but Kim noticed they were looking for a representative in her area.

Over the weekend, she mulled over the prospects. The previous fall she had taken her eldest daughter Amy, a high school senior, on a 1,900-mile trip to check out colleges in the New England area. "It was a great last fling together," Kim recalls. "I loved visiting the schools with her and seeing all the kids and what was happening on campus. It had been 20 years since I had been in college, and it was great fun to go back."

Though that trip constituted Kim's closest experience in relation to the admissions job advertised in the newspaper, by Monday she had decided to apply for it. "My daughter had collected hundreds of college catalogues at that point, so I went up to her room and started searching for one from that school. Sure enough, I soon found it, looked up the name of the director of admissions, and decided to call him directly. He is a very busy man, but he happened to be in when I called and I got to talk to him. I guess it was fate."

By this time the school had received more than 400 applications for the position, but the director arranged for Kim to meet with an admissions officer who was to be near her home that week. After passing that preliminary interview, she was invited to the campus.

"When they called and asked me up, I just said sure, without even thinking about the fact that I would be driving to New Hampshire by myself in the middle of the winter. Well, I made it there all right and checked into a little inn, very quaint and charming. Then I woke up the next day and found two feet of snow on the ground." Kim managed to hike over to the admissions office and found her efforts rewarded when she was offered the job.

"I knew I could do the job, and in the end I guess I got it because I had this confidence—cockiness almost. With four teenagers of my own, I knew I could talk to other kids, and I've always had this very strong idea about who should get into college. Basically I feel colleges should take everyone, or at least give everyone a chance. A lot of very bright kids don't do well in high school just because they've never been stimulated, turned on.

"The college I work for is a small one, and we don't go after the Ivy League recruits. Some of our students only got Cs in high school—the kind of kids whom high school counselors ordinarily send to a junior or community colege. So it's exciting to present them with the opportunity to go off to a four-year, out-of-state school.

"I'm really enthusiastic about a lot of things at the college, but I don't

"I know I should
take better care
of my skin."

try to do a big sell job on kids or their parents. The first time I went to a college night at a high school, I found myself stationed next to a recruiter who was really a huckster. He was actually trying to lure kids from my display table to his.

"Because the school I represent is not so well known, I spend a lot of time talking to guidance counselors about the place in order to determine which students might be interested in going there. It's not like recruiting for an Ivy League school, where you have kids standing in line for interviews. But I guess my job is probably more challenging.

"The nice thing about it is that I run things myself. I am not pressured to look or dress a certain way. I don't dress up too much for school interviews, but usually wear sporty clothes, skirts or pants with sweaters. Occasionally I wear suits. I set up my own appointments and choose my working hours. This still gives me time to spend on my own interests and with my children, to take them to hockey games and the dentist and things like that. And I get the summer off to be with them.

"Still, I have to do a good bit of traveling, and when I'm on the road, doing all this driving and hitting the truck stops and all that, I just wish I could be home. Working is not Nirvana.

"As far as I'm concerned, there isn't any job that's as creative as being someone's mother. The trouble is that you don't get paid for it. And that's how our society measures worth. You can raise terrific kids, but there are no external rewards, no one telling you what a great job you did. I always felt that I would go back to work sometime, get a job when the kids were grown. But they have to come first. If you don't do a decent job with them, then what's the point of anything else?"

Asked to explain her beauty routine, Kim laughs. "It's so minimal, I'm not sure it qualifies as a routine," she says. "I don't seem to be able to put makeup on so it stays, so I don't bother with it very often. I do use gel rouge, and I carry around a compact of pressed powder and a lipstick, a glossy shade. I hate the cakey kind.

I know I should take better care of my skin. It's dry and needs some help. I've seen myself age this last winter. I guess I need a moisturizer."

This diagnosis was confirmed when Kim visited Helena Rubinstein headquarters. The reason she couldn't keep makeup on very long, according to Suzanne Quinn, was because her skin was so thirsty for moisture that it was simply drinking in the emollients in the foundation. To correct this situation, Suzanne used a warm-toned moisturizer all over Kim's face before applying moisturizing makeup in a warm beige shade.

She also used eye oil wrinkle stick to dab lubrication around Kim's eye area, the part of the face that dries out most quickly. Kim had always patted a little moisturizer under her eyes and was surprised to learn that this was not a good idea. Suzanne explained that moisturizers contain water, which plumps up the skin temporarily but causes more lines when it is absorbed. It is better to use a lubricant that stays on the surface of the skin.

To hide the circles under Kim's eyes, Suzanne showed her how to pat on concealer in a shade to go with her skin tone. It is important to pat, rather than rub, so as not to stretch the skin. There is no elasticity in the under-eye area.

A ginger-colored blush was chosen for Kim's cheek color and

blended up and out toward the temples. "Oh, look where you're putting it. I never thought of that!" Kim exclaimed as it was being applied. Suzanne's advice on placing blush: Start the color no further in than the center of the eye, work out from there to emphasize cheekbones. Three tones of shadow were used on Kim's eyes: smoked teal on the lid, cool gray for contour in the crease and extended slightly beyond the corner of the eye, and sheer white for highlighting just beneath the brow bone. Next she applied smoky eyeliner in a thin line near the base of Kim's upper lashes. Brown mascara was the finishing touch for the eyes, and a touch of lipstick in a clear sienna completed the total look.

For quick touch-ups during the day when Kim is on the run, Suzanne suggested she pat more concealer lightly under her eyes and redo her cheek and lip color for an instantly fresher appearance.

Kim's dry skin needs special attention morning and night, both indoors and out: cleansing with a mild cleansing bar or a cream cleanser, toning with an alcohol-free freshener, and lots of moisturizer to protect it from the environment. Suzanne also prescribed a creamy clay mask once a week to slough off dead, dry cells and tighten and brighten the skin. She explained to Kim that the outer layer of the epidermis sheds cells in regular cycles and that every seven years our skin goes through a complete change. Since Kim is 42, she is just at the end of one cycle and starting a new one, which is why her skin had suddenly seemed different—"older"—to her.

Suzanne's final recommendations were that Kim try a neck cream at night to keep the skin on her throat firm and that she also apply an eye cream before going to bed. The eye cream could also be used during the day, in place of the eye oil wrinkle stick if Kim wanted to buy only one product. She also suggested a conditioning lash cream.

When the beauty strategy session was finished, Kim admitted that she had learned a lot and was pleasantly surprised to find that she could make changes for the better without having to spend too much time on herself.

"Sometimes I think, 'What's wrong with wrinkles?' I get them because I smile and laugh and emote a lot. They show I'm alive. On the other hand, I kid with my friends that in another couple of years we'll all check into a hospital and get our faces lifted together. One day I decide I'll just let my hair stay brown, then the next I put more blonde streaks in it. It's crazy."

How did Kim's teenagers react to their mother's more youthful look? "Kids are funny," says Kim. "They want you to look like a Mom. I think they're happiest when I look sort of dowdy ... but I think I looked terrific!"

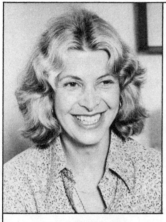

KIM DREZNER

Age: 42
Eyes: Brown
Hair: Streaked Blonde

Skin Type: Dry
Recommended Skin Care:
   Cleansing: cream cleanser or mild soap
     eye makeup remover
   Toning: alcohol-free freshener
   Day Care: moisturizer (warm shade)
     eye oil wrinkle stick
   Night Care: night cream
     eyelash cream
     eye cream
     neck cream
Special care: creamy mask

Skin Tone: Medium complexion
  with a basically facial tone
Recommended Makeup:
   Moisturizing Makeup: warm beige
   Cheek Color: ginger
   Concealer: medium
   Lip Color: clear sienna
   Lid Color: smoky teal
   Pressed Powder Eyeshadow:
     cool gray/sheer white
   Eyeliner: charcoal gray
   Lash Color: brown
   Shadow Base

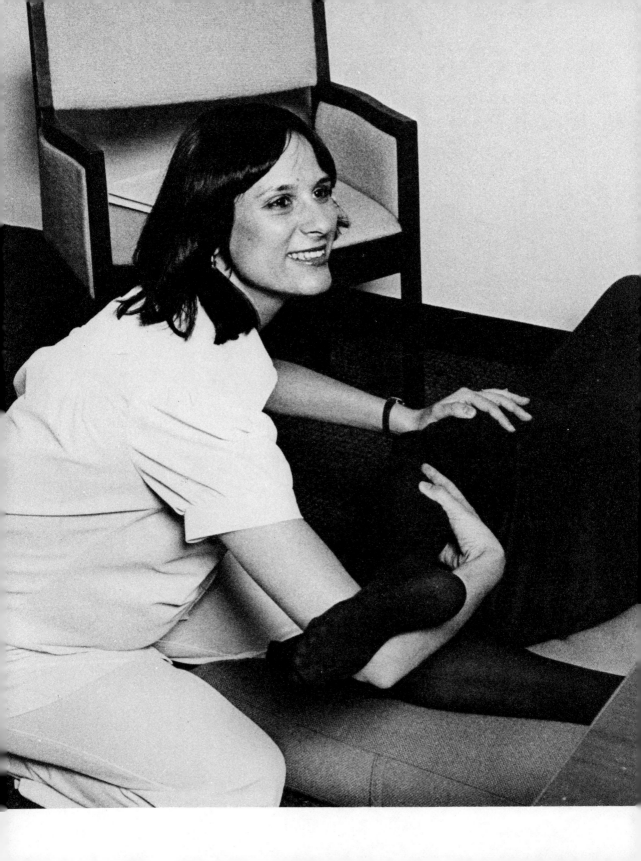

CHAPTER SIX

Standing Out in a Uniform

SUBJECT: ELLEN BODNER, PHYSICAL THERAPIST

Ellen Bodner automatically stands out in her hospital uniform these days. Several months pregnant, she can't help it. Her patients in physical therapy sometimes worry about all the bending and lifting she does while exercising their limbs, but Ellen brushes their comments aside. "I'm fine. I'm fine," is her standard response, and, indeed, in these days when it is becoming increasingly common for women to work straight through to the end of their pregnancies, Ellen is a glowingly healthy example of the reasons why. Despite the added bulk to her front side, she is as agile and chipper as ever.

"I regard pregnancy as a totally healthy experience," she says. "I don't see why I shouldn't work." Such an attitude is an expression of both her personal and professional convictions, not only as a physical therapist but as a certified Lamaze instructor. One night a week she teaches classes in her home to expectant parents preparing for childbirth. Recently she added an extra pupil, her husband Gershon.

Ellen sees her two jobs as being different, yet connected. "As I was growing up, I wanted to be a professional dancer," she says. "But when I was 18 I was in a car accident that left me temporarily paralyzed and with a broken arm. Recovering from that, I became interested in dance therapy and decided I wanted to do something where I could use the attributes of creative movement to help the physically disabled. That's how I ended up as a physical therapist. Becoming a Lamaze teacher came out of an interest in healthy people, but the breathing techniques I teach for use in labor and delivery stem from physical therapy. It's just a different application."

Ellen obtained a B.S. in science, an M.S. in educational psychology and a certificate in physical therapy. At age 27, she has worked as a therapist in the pediatrics department of a large metropolitan hospital for three-and-one-half years.

Ellen teaches group classes at the hospital and also works individually with eight to 10 patients a day, all of them ranging in age from one year to 17. Her usual workday starts at 9 A.M. with "ambulation" class. Half a dozen children in wheelchairs are lined up in a long room equipped with a set of parallel bars and a three-way mirror at one end. One by one, Ellen lifts the children from their wheelchairs and helps them practice walking with crutches or by holding on to the bars. It is not an easy task, for the children or for Ellen. The young ones, in particular, are easily distracted from what she is trying to teach them.

"Are you carrying those crutches around like pocketbooks, or are you going to use them?" Ellen asks a little dark-haired girl. "Come on. Let's go to the mirrors. Crutch, step, crutch, step."

The little girl's attention wanders around the room, and she drops one of the crutches. "You see?" says Ellen. "What are you going to do now?" As she retrieves the crutch, the child complains it is too big. "If you stand up tall, it won't be," says Ellen firmly. "Let me see you stand like a nice tall girl. Where is your face?" she asks, tilting the child's head up to look at her.

After ambulation class comes the "infant stimulation" program. Ellen goes down the hall to pick up an 18-month-old child with a chromosomal imbalance that has left her mentally retarded. They return to the exercise room where Ellen and a student nurse place the baby on a mat for a developmental test, trying to get the child to follow objects and reach for toys. Ellen taps the child's shoulders to urge her toward a toy: "Come on, Val. Come on, sweetie. You can get it." Slowly a small hand reaches out, but drops to the mat before finding the object. "You wouldn't think to look at her that there's been much progress, but there has," says Ellen. "A great amount."

Next, they place the baby on her stomach and try to get her to turn over. There is no response. "The rolling today is not up to par," says Ellen. She then places the child on her hands and knees and coaxes her to crawl. The child collapses to the mat. As Ellen leans over her, the baby reaches out and touches Ellen's hair. "That's funny," says the student nurse. "She was actually focusing on you for a moment. She doesn't usually do that."

And so the day goes, full of large frustrations and small rewards. In the afternoon Ellen makes rounds in the hospital to exercise the limbs of immobilized patients. One such is Mary, an 11-year-old who has suffered a brain tumor and is comatose. Gently Ellen lifts the girl's arms and legs, stretching and flexing them carefully. "I put her through a range of motions to keep her joints loose so that if her condition improves she can walk." The girl's mother comes into the room, and

"I always wear
make up to work.
It makes me
feel brighter to
have some color
on my face."

Ellen demonstrates the procedures to her, so that she will be able to do them when the child is able to go home. After making her rounds, there are still reports that she must fill out on each of her patients and sometimes meetings to attend. By 4:30, Ellen's busy workday is finally over.

Does it bother her, being pregnant, to work with children who have so many disabilities and impairments? "Sometimes I worry—I suppose all pregnant women do—about whether my baby will be healthy," she says. "But I remind myself that I'm healthy, and there's no reason to anticipate that anything will go wrong. Toward the end of the pregnancy I'll be doing therapy on adult outpatients rather than the children, simply because at that point I won't be able to lift the kids and carry them around."

Will she return to work after she has her baby? "Definitely, at some point. I'm just not sure when. I'm taking the maternity leave the hospital offers and then, well, we'll see."

●

Being pregnant has necessitated a few adjustments in Ellen's regular schedule. For instance, she cut her usual mile of jogging at 5:30 A.M. to a half mile a day and decided to give it up altogether in her fifth month. She has also curtailed her after-work dance classes, though she continues to do her own stretching and mobility exercises at home to music. "Dancing used to be my release," she says. "Now when I want to unwind, I'm more likely to stretch out in bed with a good book. I'm still a pretty early riser. I like to have plenty of time in the morning to shower and get ready for work."

She estimates that she spends about half an hour on her morning routine, which besides a shower consists of applying liquid foundation, blusher, lip gloss, mascara, and shadow. "I always wear makeup to work. It makes me feel brighter to have some color on my face."

When Ellen had her session at Helena Rubinstein headquarters, Suzanne Quinn suggested that a bronze or mauve-colored blusher would work well with the white uniform Ellen wears at work, and that a lipstick with a pink tone would give her face the brightest look. Because Ellen's skin has a tendency toward sallowness, a warm-toned moisturizer was recommended, to be followed by foundation in a warm tawny shade. Suzanne also showed Ellen how to apply a darker foundation in a triangular-shaped area to de-emphasize her slightly prominent chin.

Ellen, like many working women, has a problem keeping her makeup fresh all day, particularly after workouts with her patients. Suzanne made two suggestions to her. First, after Ellen washes her face in the morning, with a water activated face wash or mild soap, she can apply blotting lotion in a color-corrective warm-toned shade to the oily areas around her nose, chin, and forehead. This will provide oil control to keep skin looking fresh and shine free. At the same time, moisturizer on her drier cheek area will provide a good base for foundation there. Then, after applying foundation, a light dusting of loose powder in a transparent tone will "set" the makeup and keep it looking clean longer.

To keep eye makeup in place, Suzanne applied cream shadow to

Ellen's lid and under her brow, and then smudged a walnut lid color at the base of the lashes, rather than eyeliner. A brown-toned shadow was used in the crease of the lid, extending out slightly beyond the corner of the eye. For variety, Ellen could choose a gray or gray-blue shadow for day, though Suzanne recommended staying away from any definite color.

For care of her partly dry, partly oily skin, an astringent facial mask, a product Ellen had never tried before, was prescribed for use all over the face two or three times per week. Suzanne also suggested Ellen get into the habit of using a lightweight cream along with eye cream before bed. Even though Ellen is young, Suzanne stressed that it was not too soon to start preventive measures against aging skin.

While there isn't much time for touch-ups at work, Ellen does stop off at her hospital locker at lunchtime to check her lip gloss and blusher. To keep blusher on a long time, Suzanne suggested using a cream formulation topped by a dusting of powder blush.

Ellen usually totes her own lunch from home—a sandwich, fruit or cut-up vegetables, cheese and milk—and eats it in the hospital cafeteria. Since she must be back on the job within an hour, there really isn't enough time to go out to a restaurant.

After work, Ellen occasionally meets her husband for dinner or the theater. However, since he is working on his Ph.D. while holding down a full-time job, there isn't much opportunity for such excursions these days. When they can manage the time on weekends, the Bodners go antiquing in winter or to the beach in summer. They enjoy sailing and are thinking of buying a boat.

Ellen and Gershon met the summer he painted her parents' house. As he finished one room and then another, he began to notice something peculiar. In each room, he had to remove the same portrait of a pretty, dark-haired girl from the wall. After taking down the picture for the umpteenth time, his curiosity was sufficiently aroused to ask who the girl was—the question Ellen's mother had been waiting for all along.

Ellen's makeup session at Helena Rubinstein took place the same day Gershon finished his graduate program. As they toasted in celebration, Ellen asked him how he liked her "new" face. He was enthusiastic about the results, but couldn't resist adding that he had always thought her pretty as a picture.

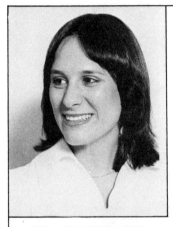

ELLEN BODNER

Age: 27
Eyes: Brown
Hair: Black

Skin Type: Partly dry, partly oily
Recommended Skin Care:
    Cleansing: water activated face wash
       or mild soap
       eye makeup remover
    Toning: toner astringent
    Day Care: moisturizer (warm shade)
       blotting lotion (warm shade)
       eye oil wrinkle stick
    Night Care: lightweight cream
       eyelash cream
       eye cream
       neck cream
Special care: astringent facial mask
Skin Tone: Medium to deep complexion
    with a basically cool tone
Recommended Makeup:
    Foundation: warm tawny
    Cheek Color: bronze or mauve
    Concealer: medium
    Loose Face Powder: transparent tone
    Lip Color: candy apple or mocha
    Lid Color: walnut or smoky slate
    Pressed Powder Eyeshadow: gray/sterling
       silver/ginger/apricot
    Lash Color: black
    Shadow Base

PART TWO

**Creating A
Working
Beauty
Routine**

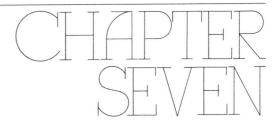

Analyzing Your Personal Needs

In Part I of this book, we studied the beauty needs of six working women and came up with routines and ideas to help them look and feel their best at their respective jobs. In this second section, the aim is to help you in the same way. We'll offer suggestions and provide step-by-step instructions to help you devise your own routine, based on your own special needs.

The first step in putting yourself together—attractively and professionally—is to know what resources you have to work with. You need a basic rundown on all those good things in bottles and tubes and wands at the cosmetics counter, so you can understand what they are, how to use them, and what they can and can't do for you.

BEAUTY TERMINOLOGY

When you buy anything, it helps to be an informed consumer. That goes for beauty products, too. To know what you're reading on product labels and package inserts, here is some basic terminology you should be familiar with:

EPIDERMIS. The outer layer of skin, the one that you can see. The epidermis is continuously sloughing off and being replaced.

ACID MANTLE. Film that covers the epidermis and keeps bacteria out. Harsh alkali soap can remove this protection.

PORES. Tiny openings in the skin through which fluids may be absorbed or discharged.

TISSUE FLUIDS. Source of all nourishment and natural moisture in the skin.

LUBRICANT. Makes skin smoother, more pliable. Also traps moisture in the skin to protect it from the environment.

EMOLLIENT. A preparation that lubricates the skin and produces a soft, smooth feeling by flattening the rough scales on the epidermis.

EMULSION. A mixture of two or more liquids that do not normally dissolve in each other—for example, oil and water. Emulsions are heavier than emollients, geared toward drier skin types.

HUMECTANT. Substance or ingredient that helps skin retain moisture and also attracts moisture from the environment.

pH VALUE. The degree of acidity or alkalinity, rated on a scale from 1 to 14. Because skin is generally slightly acidic, 7.0 is considered a neutral point in cosmetics. Higher numbers indicate alkalinity; lower numbers, acidity.

TREATMENT PRODUCTS

With the above definitions in mind, your next step is to become familiar with the different products on the market so you'll know what is available. Before getting into makeup, let's examine beauty treatments, those items designed to help you keep your skin in the best possible condition. Here's a list of treatment products and what they are used for.

SOAPS. The soaps sold at cosmetics counters are mild and specially formulated for different skin types. Because they are so gentle, they can give a soap-and-water cleansing without leaving skin feeling taut and uncomfortable. Regular soaps are alkaline and too drying for most skins past age 22 or so.

CLEANSERS. These products come in cream or lotion forms and loosen dirt and makeup so they can be tissued off. Some are water soluble, which means they should be rinsed off just like soap. Cleansers can be used as an alternative to soap or as a preliminary step to soap-and-water cleansing.

SCRUBBING GRAINS. A gritty, mildly abrasive type of cleanser that helps slough off the uppermost layer of dead skin and dirt. Grains should not be used more than once or twice a week.

ASTRINGENTS. These are liquids made from a combination of alcohol, water, and glycerin, used to cool and freshen the skin and temporarily tighten pores. Also good for quick makeup removal between regular cleansings.

FRESHENERS OR TONERS. Basically the same as astringents, these lotions contain less alcohol and so are better choices for dry or sensitive skin.

BLOTTING LOTIONS. Used under makeup, these lotions control oiliness and protect vital moisture, helping to keep skin fresh and shine free. Usually available in clear or color-corrective tones that take the ruddiness out of a too pink skin or warm a pale or sallow complexion.

MOISTURIZERS. These also make a good base for makeup or can be used alone to soothe and soften the skin. A combination of oil and water, moisturizers deposit a light film that slows down the evaporation of natural moisture and forms a protective barrier between skin and the environment.

NIGHT CREAMS. Basically the same as moisturizers, but of a heavier consistency. Special creams for the eye and neck areas have a higher concentration of oil, since these skin areas are lacking in natural oil glands.

WRINKLE STICKS. Solid lubricants that come in a lipstick-size tube. Handy to slick on during the day around the eyes and mouth for extra protection from dryness and chapping.

EYE MAKEUP REMOVERS. These come in a variety of forms: stick, gel, oil, or cream. They clean away mascara, shadow, and liner without damaging the delicate tissues of the eye area.

LASH CREAMS. Just like your hair, your eyelashes need conditioning. Available in automatic, mascara-type dispensers, these emollients roll on to give a little TLC to brittle lashes.

FACIAL MASKS. Masks freshen and tone the skin by helping slough off dry, dead surface cells, leaving a finer finish. Ingredients in masks vary. Oily skin types should use an astringent-type mask two or three times a week to control excess oil and unclog and refine pores. Dry or delicate skins should use a creamier formulation just once a week to brighten skin without drying. Masks come in cream form that is massaged into the skin, then rinsed off, or in brush-on formulas that harden into a thin latex film that is peeled off the face after it has set.

SKIN TYPES

Now that you know what treatment products are available, you need to analyze your skin type so you can make appropriate selections. One way to determine what kind of skin you have is to take a blot test. First, wash your face thoroughly, making sure to remove all traces of makeup. Then, at half-hour intervals, take a piece of ordinary white tissue paper or one layer of tissue and press it to the center of your forehead and down your nose. If you see an oil spot on the tissue the first time you try, your skin is oily. You will probably notice a difference in gloss between where you blotted and the rest of your face. If it takes an hour or so for an oil spot to develop, your skin is about normal. With dry skin you will have difficulty seeing any spot, even a couple of hours after cleansing.

Here are some recommendations from Helena Rubinstein skin-care experts on how to take the best care of your face, based on the kind of skin you have.

OILY SKIN

Oily skin is a problem of adolescence that some of us never outgrow. Yet it is a blessing in disguise. While oily skin needs special care to control breakouts and clogged pores, it is also more self-moisturizing than dry skin and thus tends to age more slowly. Fine lines often do not show up until much later in life. Here are the products you need and the steps you should take to care for your oily skin:

CLEANSE. For a soap-and-water cleansing that doesn't leave your skin feeling taut and uncomfortable, use a gentle **soap** specially formulated for oily skin types. If you like a **lotion cleanser,** choose one that can be rinsed off. You don't want heavy lubricants or an oily residue to mask your fresh clean face. Use lotion cleanser by itself or in combination with soap and water.

REFRESH AND TONE. A good **astringent** is a must for oily skin. You can't stop your system from secreting oil, but you can and should keep it from building up on the surface of your skin, where it can cause trouble. After cleansing, wipe on astringent with a cotton pad, giving special attention to the problem areas of your face: nose, chin, and forehead. Avoid the eye area.

MOISTURIZE. Oily skin needs moisture, just like drier complexions. What it doesn't need are heavy, greasy lotions to clog it and mask its appearance. **Blotting lotion** is ideal because it provides maximum oil control while giving your skin the specialized moisture protection it needs. Available in clear or color-corrective tones, blotting lotion keeps skin looking fresh and shinefree for hours. At night you'll want a **lightweight moisturizer.** See Chapter 15 for special nighttime skin-care instructions.

PARTLY DRY, PARTLY OILY SKIN

Partly dry, partly oily or, as it is usually called, combination skin consists of oily patches on the nose, chin, and forehead and dry areas on the cheeks. Many women with this type of skin try to follow two separate regimens and get bogged down in a maze of products. That

isn't necessary if you use light, nongreasy products that won't aggravate
the oil problem and at the same time will provide moisture protection
to the entire face. Here are some recommended products and directions
to care for combination skin:

CLEANSE. Many **soaps** will be too harsh and drying for your face, so
be sure to choose an extremely mild one. If your skin feels taut after
washing, change to a gentler soap. If you prefer a **lotion cleanser,** use
the rinse-off type, as you don't want heavy lubricants leaving an oily
residue. Use cleansers as an alternative to soap or as a prelude to
soap-and-water washing.

REFRESH AND TONE. You are seeking oil control for your nose,
chin, and forehead (the T zone), yet your drier cheeks need toning
and brightening, too. So just this once, you need two separate products. After cleansing and every time you change makeup, saturate a
cotton pad with **astringent** and wipe it over your T zone, avoiding the
eye area. Then apply **toner** in the same way to your cheeks, to gently
stimulate the skin without stripping it of moisture.

MOISTURIZE. The dual demands of your skin for oil control and
moisture are especially urgent during the day when you are wearing
makeup. **Blotting lotion** provides oil control as it adds and protects
vital moisture. It keeps skin looking fresh and shine free and is
available in clear or color-corrective tones. At night choose a **lightweight moisturizer** to put on your face; a heavy lubricant is the last
thing you want. See Chapter 15 for directions for nighttime care.

NORMAL TO SLIGHTLY DRY SKIN

Lucky you. All your normal to slightly dry skin needs to keep it looking its best is a good maintenance routine. By and large, your skin has few problems, and any spot dryness is probably the result of environmental stress, such as extremely warm or cold weather, or atmospheric dryness. Here are the products that will help maintain your skin's ideal balance and the steps you should take in using them:

CLEANSE. Use the mildest of **soaps** morning and night to clear and refine your skin. Rinse with warm water. If you wish, you can alternate this routine with using **cream cleanser**. A cream formulation will remove makeup gently without harmful scrubbing. Massage it lightly over face and throat, then tissue or rinse off.

REFRESH AND TONE. Whether you're wiping away the last traces of cream cleanser or putting a little zing into your skin tone, a mild yet brisk **toner** is right for your skin type. To remove cleanser traces, saturate a cotton pad with toner and run it over the area you've just cleansed. To tone, brighten, and refine, saturate another cotton pad and pat it lightly but purposefully on face and throat. Avoid eye area.

MOISTURIZE. Choose a **lightweight moisturizer** to wear alone or under makeup by day. At night you could use a **moisturizing emulsion** or, if your skin has been exposed to harsh conditions, a **lightweight cream moisturizer.** See Chapter 15 for more about nighttime care.

DRY TO VERY DRY SKIN

If you were to think of your skin type as a flower, it would have to be considered a hothouse variety—beautiful but frail, vulnerable to the slightest whim of your environment. Your skin reacts swiftly to changes in the weather, central heating and cooling units, even to pollution. It chaps easily in winter, turns painfully red after minutes of sun exposure, is constantly thirsting for moisture. Here are the products and special care instructions you need for your delicate dry skin:

CLEANSE. It was once thought that heavy cream cleansers were the only option for dry skin, but no more. The **mild soaps** specially formulated for dry skin are so gentle that you can use them morning and night. Wash with warm water only, as extreme hot or cold temperatures are too hard on your fragile skin. Alternate, if you like, with a **cream cleanser,** to remove makeup gently without scrubbing. Massage cleanser lightly over face and throat, then tissue away or rinse off.

REFRESH AND TONE. Dry to very dry skin can often look listless and pale. It needs a gentle stimulant to perk up its appearance and remove the dead surface cells that mask its clarity. Choose an **alcohol-free toner** for its mild ingredients and skin-soothing emollients. Saturate a cotton pad with toner and smooth it over your face and throat using upward strokes. Your skin should feel soothed and cooled, but not dry.

MOISTURIZE. Your skin is always thirsty and, what's more, it is constantly losing moisture. Whether or not you wear makeup, you need a moisturizer. For daytime, smooth a **moisturizing emulsion** over your face and throat, wait about 30 seconds to let your skin drink it up, then apply your makeup. This will not only protect your skin, but help keep your makeup looking fresh. If you're not wearing makeup, the moisturizing emulsion will act as a layer of protection from the weather outside or a centrally heated room. A **night cream** is a must for very dry skin. About 20 minutes before bedtime, smooth it over your freshly cleansed face, using upward motions. If you prefer a fluffier consistency, you could also choose a **lightweight cream** and alternate the two to give your skin a nice balance, especially at times when it is not so dry. See Chapter 15 for more special nighttime instructions.

COSMETIC PRODUCTS

Now that you know the right treatment products and routines to use with your skin type, you are ready to select makeup. This gets a little more complicated, because not only do you need to choose formulations that are right for your kind of skin, but you must match colors with your eyes, hair, and skin tone. Before getting into coloring, here is a rundown of various makeup products and what they can do for you.

FOUNDATION. Properly selected and applied, foundation can give skin a finer texture, even out its natural coloring, and conceal minor imperfections. For the most natural look, choose a shade that closely matches your own skin tone. There are different formulations for different skin types. Choose a rich, sheer emollient for dry to very dry skin, a balanced formula for normal to slightly dry skin, and a water-based, long-lasting formula for oily and combination skin.

CONCEALER. Available in cream or stick form, concealer helps cover under-eye shadows, small splotches, and blemishes. Choose a shade just a bit lighter than your foundation color. If you don't wear foundation, choose a shade to match your skin tone.

BLUSHER. Blusher colors and contours the face. Applied correctly, it should give you a natural, healthy glow. Generally, a powdered blush works better for oily skin, while a cream blush is best for drier skin types. Use gel blushers sparingly, as they dry quickly and can streak.

FACE POWDER. Without a finishing touch of powder, makeup attracts and holds dirt from the air. It smears more easily and doesn't last as long. Powder comes in two forms, pressed and loose. The loose form should be dusted lightly over foundation to set it. The pressed form can be used later in the day for touch-ups without smearing.

MASCARA. This is considered by many women to be their one indispensable cosmetic item. Select a mascara color close to the color of your own lashes. Too dark mascara or a heavy hand in application make for an unnatural effect. Some formulas are water resistant (so they stay on till you remove them); others have special conditioners to keep your lashes from becoming dry or brittle, and have to be reapplied during the day.

EYELINER. To help define eyes, you can use eyeliner at the base of your lashes. For best results, stroke color on with a fine pencil or brush, then smudge with your fingertip. You do not want an obvious line ringing your eyes.

EYESHADOW. Shadow further accentuates the eyes, but must be used very subtly during the day. For office hours, choose neutral tones—browns, grays, taupes—for lid color. **Highlighter,** which is used under the curve of the brow, should be in light warm tones—pale pink, beige, sand—by day. For evening wear, you can go all out, with deep colors, silvers, and golds. Shadows come in powder or cream forms; experiment to find which works best for you.

LIP COLORS. Lip colors come in a range of formulations: cream, frost, and translucent lipsticks, as well as clear and colored glosses. Besides coloring, they help keep lips from becoming dry and chapped. Pale lips need brightening for a healthy look; if you have natural color, you could just choose a clear gloss to protect and moisturize. Using color and a lip brush for precise application, it is possible to make minor corrections in the shape of your lips, making thin lips appear fuller and vice versa.

SKIN TONES

It is not possible to prescribe exact choices for makeup colors in a book. You really need to visit a cosmetics counter and use the testers to see how certain shades will look on you. Don't just look at the color in the bottle or tube and hope it will be right. Consult with the cosmetician, if you need advice. Here are some general tips from Helena Rubinstein makeup experts for different skin tones:

LIGHT TO MEDIUM COMPLEXION WITH A BASICALLY WARM TONE. You want to try to tone down the extra pinkness in your skin and even out its overall color. Your foundation choices range from cool ivory to cool bisque to cool beige. If you have widespread areas of ruddiness (as in the cheek area), choose a makeup that is one tone deeper than your natural skin shade. It makes the cover-up easier. By bringing your skin tone closer to beige, you open up a range of other color possibilities. You can then wear even the new neutral shades—

taupes, browns, etc.—which otherwise would not be that flattering for you.

MEDIUM TO DEEP COMPLEXION WITH A BASICALLY WARM TONE. Your goal is to tone down the ruddiness in your skin, even out its overall tone and bring it closer to beige. Your foundation choices range from cool beige to cool tawny to cool amber. If you are covering widespread areas of ruddiness, it is better to choose the deepest available shade and blend it out carefully. By bringing your skin tone closer to beige, it is possible for you to wear even the so-called naturals—beiges and taupes—which heretofore looked muddy on you.

LIGHT TO MEDIUM COMPLEXION WITH A BASICALLY BALANCED TONE. Since your skin is neither too pink nor too yellow, all you have to do is enhance your good fortune. Your foundation options include six different shades: warm or cool ivories, bisques, and beiges. Since you have no corrections to make, let your wardrobe determine whether you use a cool or warm shade. With blue, pink, plum, or blue-green, wear the cool range. For rusts, golds, naturals and fire-engine red, use warm tones.

MEDIUM TO DEEP COMPLEXION WITH A BASICALLY BALANCED TONE. You have no major corrections to make in your skin tone, since there are no outstanding casts of pink, yellow, or olive. Your foundation choices include six different shades: warm or cool beiges, tawnies, and ambers. Wear cool shades with your blue, pink, and plum fashions. Switch to the warms when you wear yellows, naturals, and browns.

LIGHT TO MEDIUM COMPLEXION WITH A BASICALLY COOL TONE. You will want to correct sallow tendencies and brighten your general skin tone. Your foundation choices include warm ivory, warm bisque, and warm beige. If you find yourself undecided, it is better to choose a deeper shade over a lighter one. The important thing is that the basic tone brightens your complexion. By neutralizing your skin's yellow undertones, you can wear rosier fashion shades that otherwise wouldn't work so well for you.

MEDIUM TO DEEP COMPLEXION WITH A BASICALLY COOL TONE. You will want to brighten your appearance and correct your skin's tendency to sallowness. Your foundation choices range from warm beige to warm tawny to warm amber. If you find yourself undecided, opt for the deeper shade. All will neutralize sallowness and add life to your coloring. By correcting your skin's yellow undertones, you will find you can even wear pink, ordinarily not one of your best shades.

After reading this chapter, you may decide you need to make a shopping expedition to stock the right products for your skin type and coloring. If so, be sure to consult the cosmetician at the beauty counter. Some women hesitate to do so, for fear they'll be talked into buying a lot of products they don't need. But this shouldn't worry you. A good salesperson is interested in having you as a repeat customer, so she isn't likely to recommend products that you won't be satisfied with or will feel are a waste of money. Besides, advice is free and should be given readily, whether or not you intend to make any purchases. You are under no obligation and can simply walk away if you feel you are being pressured.

At several cosmetics counters in big department stores, you'll now find instant "beauty analyzers," quick and foolproof systems to help you select the right makeup and treatment products. These are actual electronic computer operations based on different hair colors, eye colors, and skin tones, from very pale to brown and deep olive.

By answering some simple questions, you feed your skin tone, hair, and eye color to the analyzer, which makes a composite picture and issues you an identity number. You can then press the corresponding button on a makeup tester bar, and like magic the correct products for your type will light up so you can try them right on the spot.

The skin-care section of the analyzer works the same way. You answer more questions, are issued an identity number, then feed that number to the skin-care tester. The products to use in a regimen that's best for your skin type will light up. The whole process takes only minutes and is a real boon to the busy working woman.

Once you have the right basic resources, it is much easier to organize a quick and efficient beauty routine to use throughout your day.

CHAPTER EIGHT

Devising a Quick and Easy Morning Routine

Do you ever start your day on the verge of hysteria because you don't have a single blouse ironed or because the skirt you wanted to wear has a nice big spot on it? Ever want to scream when you can't locate your lipstick or that hairbrush you had in your hand only a second ago? Are you so busy trying to get some food in front of a husband and/or child that you're lucky to end up with a coffee and Danish at the office yourself? Do you always seem to be missing buses or trains, thereby arriving at work harried and frazzled and feeling as though you've already put in a full day?

You can call a halt to all this, if you are willing to do a little advance planning. Organization is the key, plus some practical remedial measures. But it *is* possible to keep your mornings under control and start your working day a new person. Chances are, you won't be able to break all your old habits overnight. But you can certainly begin making things easier on yourself. A certain amount of discipline is required, but it will more than pay off in the way you end up looking and feeling once you are into your new routine.

CHARTING YOUR TIME

To begin at the beginning, take a few moments to figure out how much time you generally give yourself between the time you wake up and the time you must be out the door. Fifteen minutes? Half an hour? An hour? How many things do you have to accomplish during this time? Besides getting yourself up and dressed, how many other family members are you responsible for? How many breakfasts do you have to make? What other chores like bed making or dog walking take up your time?

If you are sincerely interested in getting organized, it would be a good idea to sit down and actually compile a list of all the routine things you do each morning. Don't forget to include brushing your teeth or setting your hair with electric rollers. Next to each listing, make a *reasonable* estimate of how long it should take you to do each item: washing face (three minutes), putting on makeup (five minutes), etc. Now total. How does this figure compare with the amount of time you are presently allotting yourself? Note: You should probably add at least an extra 15 minutes "transition time" to your final figure to take into account minutes spent moving from one activity to another and to allow for the usual foul-ups.

Say you have just discovered that your morning duties take one hour and 10 minutes and you have only been allotting 45. One of the choices you have is to get up 25 minutes earlier each morning. If you can't bear that thought, you have to either cut down the time you spend on some activities or cut them out altogether. Consider, for instance,

—washing your hair the night before, so you don't have to worry

about getting it dry in the morning;
—laying out your clothes ahead of time so you know what is clean
   and which items are missing buttons;
—packing lunches in advance;
—having your husband get the kids' breakfast;
—getting a no-fuss hairstyle that just needs a quick comb-through;
—leaving the beds unmade.

LARKS AND OWLS

Perhaps you think it would just be easier to get up a half hour earlier. However, if you aren't a "morning person," you may need help getting out of bed. Basically, there are two kinds of people in this world, larks and owls. Larks arise chipper and eager to get about their business. Owls take a peek at the new day and burrow deeper under the covers. Extreme owl cases don't hit their stride until midnight or so, long after the larks have called it a day. Unfortunately, the business world pretty much functions on the larks' schedule. And owls must accommodate.

Since getting up in the morning can be painful enough in itself, don't add to your miseries with a jangling alarm clock. It may get you out of bed, but it will probably shatter your nerves, not to mention a great dream, in the process. You would be better off investing in a clock radio, which will wake you up a little more soothingly but still not allow you to slip back off to sleep. Put the radio across the room—not next to your bed where you will be tempted to switch it off—and remember to adjust the volume to a bit louder than normal.

When the radio goes off in the morning, you don't have to stumble out of bed immediately. Take a few moments to yawn and stretch while you're still lying down. Open your mouth wide and take in as much air as you can. Stretch your legs out and try to touch the bottom of the bed with your toes. Put your arms up in the air and reach for the ceiling. Now swing your legs to the floor and sitting on the edge of the bed, reach down toward your toes. Hang there for just a moment, then sit up straight. Hunch your shoulders up to your ears, then relax. Repeat a couple of times. You should now have some of the overnight kinks worked out and be ready to get on your feet.

Once you're up, keep moving. Walk around the kitchen rather than slumping into a chair. Rise up on your toes a few times while you brush your teeth. NEVER get back into bed, no matter how tempting another few moments in the sack may be. If you can stand food at this point, it always helps to get a little nourishment into your body.

ABOUT BREAKFAST

Everyone should eat something for breakfast. If the sight or thought of food is less than appealing when you first get up, make sure you have something to eat when you get to the office. Walking to work, at least part of the way, followed by an energizing breakfast at your desk is an excellent way to get yourself revved up for the day.

Even if you ate a late dinner the night before, your body will still have gone many hours without food and will need to be refueled. Many people who don't wake up hungry think they can lose weight by skipping breakfast. But studies have shown that obese people are more likely to be breakfast skippers (they make up for it by overeating later in the day), while breakfast eaters tend to maintain a balanced weight. In order to give you a sufficient amount of energy to carry you through the morning, breakfast should contain protein and carbohydrates. The energy available in various food components is released at different times, depending on how long it takes to digest. You'll get a boost from carbohydrates first, from proteins later on.

The typical office breakfast of coffee and a sweet roll (some 275 calories) is almost as bad as skipping breakfast altogether. You will get a temporary energy rush from the sugar, but it will wear off quickly, leaving you feeling more dragged out than before. Coffee does nothing for you nutritionally and too much caffeine (if you drink cup after cup) can make you nervous and shaky.

Breakfast on the run *can* be nutritious, if you choose from the following items:

corn *or* bran muffin *or* whole-wheat toast
with
½ cup yogurt *or* ½ cup cottage cheese *or* hard-boiled egg *or* 1 cup skimmed milk *or* 1 ounce hard cheese
or
peanut butter sandwich *or* bagel with cream cheese

Eat the above with a piece of fresh fruit or fruit juice and you will have a balanced meal with protein, carbohydrates, and vitamins for about 300 calories.

At home, you can vary your repertoire with a fortified breakfast cereal (check the box for vitamin, iron, and protein listings) or poached or scrambled eggs. Authorities are still disputing whether or not you should limit your weekly intake of eggs. If you are worried about cholesterol levels, you could eat only the whites or make scrambled eggs with two whites and one yolk. The whites contain no cholesterol, only about 17 calories, and are an excellent protein source.

You can whip up a quick breakfast in a blender by combining orange juice, a raw egg, and a bit of honey. Just pour and drink. Or toss a sliced banana and some ice cubes in with an envelope of vanilla-flavored instand breakfast and skim milk for a delicious shake. If you are really, really pinched for time, grab a vitamin-fortified breakfast bar to eat on your way out the door. It's better for you than a doughnut.

GETTING READY

A few lucky people have both the time and the energy to do some exercising in the morning before work. If you jog or jump rope, you also need to schedule some extra time for showering and perhaps washing your hair. If this is your regular morning routine, you're best off having your hair cut in a wash-and-wear style so you don't damage it with too much blow-drying. The ideal cut is one that you can let dry naturally, then just shake or comb through with your fingers and be set to go. You may need a permanent to make this easy-care routine work. If you use a blow-dryer often, invest in one with adjustable temperatures and air-flow settings. Allow your hair to air-dry for 15 minutes while you dress or eat breakfast before you use the dryer. Be sure to hold it at least 10 inches from your scalp and keep it moving. Your hair may occasionally need hot oil treatments or deep conditioning to offset the drying effects of all that heat.

Whether or not you bathe or shower in the morning, you should start every day with a proper face cleansing. Using a lotion cleanser or mild soap, massage in gentle circles all over your face, concentrating especially on the T zone, the area between your brows, down your nose and around your chin, which for many women is oily. Rinse thoroughly, as soap residues can irritate your face. Use warm water: too hot and too cold are hard on the skin.

Next, splash on astringent or toner, according to your skin type, with a saturated cotton pad. Again, pay special attention to the T zone and, for those with oily skin, the hairline. Follow with a lightweight moisturizer or blotting lotion, in either clear or color-corrective tones. If you use a foundation, either of these products will help keep it looking fresh. If you don't, they provide a light covering to protect your skin from the environment. If you have dry or delicate skin, pat on all over (except eye area). If skin is oily, use only on cheeks or other areas that may be drier than the rest of your face.

Working
Woman's
Beauty
Book

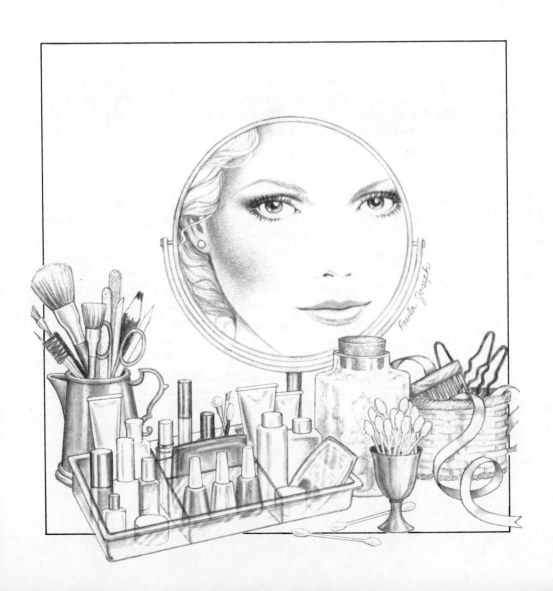

YOUR BEAUTY SPOT

The treatment routine described above can be accomplished in the bathroom in a matter of minutes. Your makeup routine needn't take much longer, but if there are others in line to use the bathroom you might want to move to another area. An essential element in keeping your routine fast and organized is to have your own spot where everything you need is right at hand. If you're stumbling over small children, or having to share half a mirror with your husband or roommate, you'll probably double the time it takes you to get ready, not to mention the irritation factor.

A bedroom dressing table needn't be the kidney-shaped, frilly-skirted affair of the past, unless that sort of thing appeals to you. You could use the top of a desk or dresser or a Parsons table made of Lucite or natural wood. The main thing is to keep it uncluttered, and have a place for everything and everything in its place. Buy Lucite canisters, little straw baskets, or apothecary jars to store such things as cotton balls, bobby pins, and cotton swabs. Cosmetic organizers, with tiers and trays, are a great idea for holding lipsticks, tubes, and brushes. For a really elegant touch, you could choose accessories in pewter or china; little bos, cups, sugars and creamers all make good stashes. Finally, you need a good-sized mirror and a strong, direct light in case you're not near a window to get the sun.

THE THREE- TO FIVE-MINUTE MAKEUP

Once you have everything you need assembled at your fingertips, makeup application shouldn't take more than three to five minutes,

particularly since your face is already clean and primed with moisturizer. Here are the next steps to take, keeping in mind that you are
using makeup to enhance your looks, not to hide them. Anything
obvious—that calls attention to the makeup rather than you—is out.
When you're done, you want to look so good that people think you're
not wearing any makeup at all, but are just naturally healthy and
glowing.

Step #1: Lubrication

The area around your eyes needs special attention, since it is
lacking in natural lubricants and can get very dry and lined. Rather
than using moisturizer here, it is a good idea to dot on eye cream or
use eye wrinkle stick, which comes in a tube like a lipstick. Dip your
ring finger into the cream or rub it across the stick, then gently pat the
lubrication under your eyes, starting at the outside corner and working your way inward toward your nose. If your lips are dry or
chapped, you can use the same oil stick to slick some lubrication on
them.

Ptep #2: Bye-Bye Bags

Many women are bothered by dark circles under their eyes, which
give a tired and older look to the face. To make these circles less
obvious, use a concealer or a foundation one shade lighter than your
skin tone. As described in the last step, pat it on very gently, and
sparingly, with your ring finger and blend evenly. The eye area is so
delicate that you never want to pull or stretch it. Always work from
the outside in.

Step #3: Base

Some women like to wear foundation and others don't. If your skin is blotchy or uneven in tone, a foundation can give a smoother look. Not everyone needs it, however. To apply, dot foundation onto your face in several spots, then blend with downward sweeping strokes. (Note: When applying makeup work in a *downward* direction, when applying treatments work *up*.) When you're through blending, pat a dry cotton ball or slightly damp washcloth over your face to remove any excess foundation.

Step #4: Concealer

If you're troubled by an occasional bump or minor breakout, you can temporarily cover the trouble spot by dotting on a little concealer in a shade to match your natural skin tone. If you're wearing foundation, use a slightly lighter shade of concealer. Choose a medicated formula, which will help heal the blemish that it hides. If frequent breakouts are a problem, consider whether you are getting enough sleep and eating a balanced diet. Consult a dermatologist for the proper treatment of problem skin.

Step #5: Powder

Whether you use foundation or not, dust on a little loose translucent powder with a puff or, better still, a big, soft brush. This will keep your makeup looking clean and fresh longer. And if you aren't wearing foundation, it will give skin a more refined texture. Dust powder over eyelashes, too, so mascara will cling better. Just don't get it into your eyes; keep them shut during the process.

Step #6: Blusher

Finding where to put cheek color is sometimes a problem if you don't have Faye Dunaway's bone structure. To find the correct spot for your face, run your fingers down your cheekbone till you reach a spot just below the middle of your eye. Put the color there and blend upward and out toward the hairline. You might also want to dab a little blusher over the bridge of your nose for a warm glow.

Step #7: Eye Shading

Skip this step unless you have the time to handle it carefully and subtly. First, to shape the eyes, draw a fine line at the base of your upper lashes in a smoky hue. Gently smudge this line with your fingertip or a cotton swab so that you don't see a definite outline. Then, if you wish to shade, use shadow in and just above the crease in your eyelid. Extend the color out past the end of the eye slightly. Again, the look should be smudged, not drawn on. Use browns or muted shadows; no turquoise, needless to say. To highlight eyes, stroke color in a line directly following the undercurve of your brow. Pale pinks, apricots, beiges, and sands are good highlighter shades for day, providing a sheen that sets off the eyes. Just be sure to blend well.

Step #8: Mascara

Apply mascara starting at the outer corner of the top lashes and working inward. Stroke on carefully from base to ends, making sure each lash is coated. Do lower lashes, too. If mascara smudges, gently rub the smudge away with a cotton swab dipped in water (eye makeup remover may make the mascara run). If any lashes are clumped together when you're finished, use an old toothbrush to separate them. For your daytime office look, one application of mascara is usually sufficient. Repeat applications, which make lashes look thicker and more lush, should be saved for special evening occasions. Remember, you want to look natural.

Step #9: Lip Color

If you have pale lips, you will probably need a lipstick with some color. If you have natural color in your lips, you may prefer to use just a colorless gloss. While glosses and frosts can give a nice, fresh look, too much sheen looks gooey. Don't overdo it. Also, unless you work in a high-fashion environment, it's probably a good idea to avoid lipstick in too bright or too deep colors. Even if the look is in vogue, it can be too noticeable and distracting. Use a soft, warm shade that will brighten the face without overpowering it.

Step #10: Scent

If you're going to wear fragrance during office hours, it should be barely perceptible. Choose a light floral, citrus, or spicy scent or one of the new designer fragrances now appearing on the market. Leave sexy musks and heavy romantic perfumes for after-work hours. Bathing with scented soap or bath gel and smoothing on body lotion in the same fragrance is a way of "layering" scent that is light but effective. As the aroma wears off, you can reinforce it with a splash of cologne at pulse points. Perfume, which is more concentrated and longer lasting, should be used sparingly by day. If someone tells you they like your perfume, you'll know you're wearing too much.

That takes care of your morning routine, and though it may seem like a lot on paper, you'll find it takes very little time in actual practice. For one thing, you probably won't be doing all 10 steps each day. For anoher, as you get into your routine it will become easier and faster as time goes by. The main thing to remember is to keep your mornings as simple, as uncluttered, and as organized as possible. You'll save a lot of unnecessary wear and tear on your sanity and get your day off to the best possible start.

CHAPTER NINE

Planning Your On-the-Job Beauty Strategy

You are up, dressed, and ready to dash out the door. All you have to do is grab your bag and run—provided you are organized enough to have everything you'll need during the day already stashed away. If you have to spend time looking for your keys or a checkbook, your quick getaway is blown.

Now that you have your morning at-home routine together, it's time to examine your workday. The first step in planning your on-the-job beauty strategy is to make sure you get out the door with everything you need. Make a mental checklist by remembering the three Ms that must be toted along to work with you each day. The first is money. You need your wallet and/or coin purse, credit-card case, and checkbook, unless you carry one of those handy combination wallets that has everything together. Next, you need makeup. It can be transported easily and neatly in one of those clear plastic zippered bags that you can buy at the dime store. You can see everything at a glance, and nothing will spill into your bag or briefcase. Third, your memos, those reminders of what you're supposed to do and where you're supposed to be and when. Always carry a pocket calendar or date book and memo pad. Be a list maker, so you don't forget errands or appointments. Also, take along an address book with frequently used phone numbers jotted inside the front cover. Not on the list of necessities, but a handy extra to carry around, is a fold-up tote bag that you can use to haul groceries, books, packages, and the like. One nylon version comes in a little zippered purse for only $5.

Once you have all your gear together, the next consideration is what sort of bag to store it in. It's handy to have one with lots of compartments, so you can find things fast. But chunky purses do not work with the snappy business look you want to maintain. An excellent idea is a canvas-and-leather portfolio with short handles and a snap-on shoulder strap. This holds a lot, yet has a sleek, tailored look. If you carry around office work and papers, you should get an actual briefcase. Some cases are roomy enough that you can slip accessories (provided they're slim) into one compartment. If you don't have room for everything, an envelope clutch is a good choice to carry with a briefcase. It's smart looking, and you can just tuck it under your arm, since you already have one hand occupied.

YOUR PORTABLE BEAUTY BAG

To make on-the-job beauty repairs, you must be well equipped. Here is a list of items that you might want to carry around in your cosmetics case:

* concealer
* wrinkle stick

* compact with mirror
* cheek color
* lipstick and/or gloss with brush
* emery board
* aspirin
* face blotters
* tissues
* hairbrush and/or comb

That is all you need to handle touch-ups. If, however, you want to redo your makeup during the day, you'll need to add

* cleanser and/or soap
* eye makeup remover
* moisturizer or blotting lotion
* bobby pins or clips
* foundation
* mascara
* shadow/highlighter
* cotton swabs
* cotton pads
* astringent or toner

Some other items that are handy, especially if you exercise at lunch hour or go out for the evening straight from work:

* deodorant
* toothbrush and toothpaste
* perfume (purse atomizer)
* barrettes or combs

This may seem like a long list, but you can probably get everything into one bag if you think small. Buy trial or travel sizes of products, or use the samples (usually miniatures) that cosmetics companies offer as gifts-with-purchase. Then, too, many of the items listed come in tubes or slim wands that take up very little space.

YOUR DESK EMERGENCY KIT

Of course, there is a limit to how much you can tote back and forth to the office each day. So it is useful to also stock a desk emergency kit. Then you'll always be prepared for on-the-job fix-ups and day-to-day disasters. The items you keep on hand will depend to some extent on the type of job you have and the amount of drawer space available, but here is a basic list:

* hand cream
* box of tissues
* towelettes or pop-up washcloths
* nail repair kit
* eyedrops
* extra pair of panty hose
* tampons

If you have enough space and can lock your desk or office, you might also want to keep:

* curling iron or portable electric rollers
* smock

* poncho or slicker
* fold-up umbrella

ON-THE-JOB BEAUTY REPAIRS

Once your portable beauty bag and desk emergency kit are assembled, you should have no trouble coping with any beauty problems that crop up. Here are some strategies to help keep you looking good:

●

If your skin is oily, but you don't have time to wash it and redo your makeup, use little linen face blotters to get rid of shine without disturbing makeup.

●

If at all possible, give your face a light once-over cleaning after lunch to remove smudges and any oiliness that may have accumulated during the morning. Go over your face with cotton pads soaked with lotion cleanser (for dry skin) or astringent (for oily skin). Reapply moisturizer or blotting lotion, and dab eye cream or wrinkle stick under your eyes. If you're wearing foundation, redo that and your cheek and lip color. You should be able to clean your face without disturbing your eye makeup, so you don't have to take time fixing that.

●

On a day when you're chairing a meeting or making a presentation,

Working
Woman's
Beauty
Book

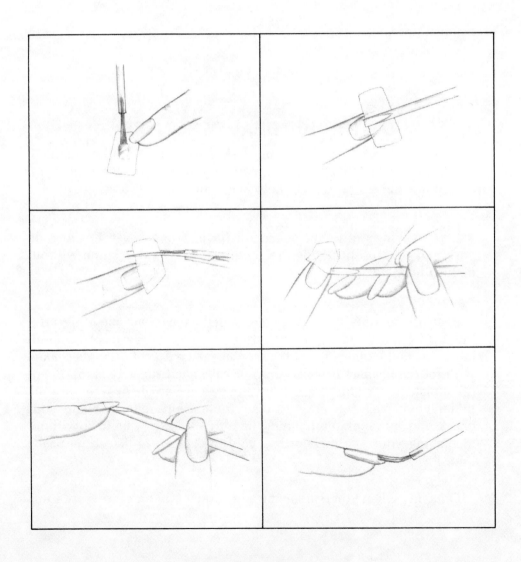

reapply your deodorant or antiperspirant during the day. Stress, not heat, activates underarm odor.

●

If you type a lot and touch carbons and ribbons, keep your hands away from your eyes, as smeary black ink is a terrible eye irritant. It's also bad for your complexion, so don't touch your face, either.

●

Keeping your hands away from your face is a good idea anyway. If you habitually rest your forehead on your fingertips or your chin in your hand, you are bringing dirt to your face and stretching the skin, which will eventually break down the natural elasticity. Hold your head up if you want to forestall wrinkles and keep your jawline firm.

●

To patch a broken nail, you need a "wrap and repair" kit. Buy one or put together your own. You need base coat, glue, orange stick, patching paper, manicure scissors, and polish (optional). Apply base coat to the nail, and put a small amount of glue on the patching paper. Drop the patch over the break, allowing enough overlap to turn under nail. Trim patch along the sides, then gently push the excess under the nail tip. Dab on more glue if necessary, then two more layers of base coat. Finish with polish if you like.

●

Take a few minutes to check your lipstick and blusher from time to time. If it's faded, reapply so you don't get a washed-out look as the day progresses.

●

If you are frequently bothered by chapped lips, it may be because you unconsciously lick them while you're busy working. Try to monitor yourself, or ask a friend to help you find out if you have a habit that needs breaking. To clear up the condition and prevent further dehydration, use a lip balm or wrinkle stick often during the day.

●

If you're doing a lot of close work, rest your eyes every 20 minutes or so by focusing on something as far away as you can see. If your eyes feel tired, place your palms directly over them and visualize black velvet. Do this for two or three minutes at a time, while releasing any tension in your neck and shoulders with the exercises described at the end of this chapter.

●

Getting to work in rainy weather without looking like you've been standing under a waterfall can be a problem. Make sure you are well protected with a full-length water-repellent coat, a rain scarf or close-fitting hat, and a good-sized umbrella. Choose a coat in a fabric that "breathes." Some vinyls don't, and you'll end up hot and perspiring by the time you get to the office. Boots are a good idea; you won't ruin a pair of shoes, and you'll protect your panty hose from splatters. If you do get mud on your hose, you can remove it quickly with a cotton ball moistened with skin toner (from your beauty bag).

If you are lucky enough to have your own office, you may be able to make your beauty repairs in private without having to scoot off to the ladies' room. Just make sure your door is shut and that you don't take too long. It's helpful to include a good-size mirror in your office decor, either a stand-up model for a shelf or bookcase, or a hanging one for the wall. Choose a mirror in an attractive wood frame to go with a traditional office; for a more modern look, select a colorful plastic. Two especially good ideas: a plastic wall organizer with a mirror and several pocket compartments to hold odds and ends; or, for a practical conversation piece, an old-fashioned wooden shaving stand. The latter wouldn't take up much space in a corner and features not only a mirror but usually a small drawer and cabinet where touch-up items can be stowed.

IMPROVING YOUR ENVIRONMENT

The lack of moisture in most centrally heated and cooled offices is bad news for your skin and thus an ongoing beauty problem. When indoor air is so dry it creates static-electric shocks and parches the nose and throat passages, it can be a health problem, too.

There are a couple things you can do to improve the situation at least partially. The most helpful step is to buy a small cold-mist humidifier and run it frequently. If you have your own office or cubicle, this should be no problem. If you're in a typing-pool arrangement, you may need to check with the people around you, or even the office manager, to see if they would mind. (Some humidifiers operate with a slight hum, which might be disturbing.) You might want to get to work early so you can run the humidifier for a little while before anyone else arrives, or plug it in during lunch hour.

A portable plastic unit can cost as little as $11; wooden consoles to blend with a plusher office decor range from about $30 to $150. The American Medical Association advises weekly washing of portable humidifiers with detergent to ensure that they are free of bacteria, which could be carried into the air. Frequent cleaning also minimizes the chance that mineral deposits from the water will clog the unit.

Another idea for the parched-air problem is to keep some plants on your desk or in your office. Not only will they give off some moisture themselves, but you can mist them daily and spritz extra water into the air. In fact, when you're feeling blah and your skin is dry, take the mister and spray your face lightly, then blot with a tissue. You'll feel refreshed and your makeup won't be disturbed.

For suggestions on plants that are a good size for a desk, will grow under office lights, and can survive weekends without watering, get hold of *The Office Gardener* by Jacqueline Heriteau (Hawthorne Books, $5.95).

You will also feel better on the job if you pay some attention to the chair you sit in. Next to your bed, this is the most important piece of furniture in your life. Most office chairs have an adjustable seat and back. So if yours is uncomfortable, don't squirm—do something about it. Sometimes you can make height adjustments easily by using a lever underneath the seat. If your chair is more complicated, call the office manager. The proper height for the backrest is at the shoulder blades. The right height for the seat allows you to sit comfortably with both feet flat on the floor. If the seat is too high, there will be pressure on the undersides of the thighs, which over a period of time could result in circulation problems.

The small of your back (the lower lumbar region) should fit snugly into the chair back, which should be slightly convex to accommodate the natural bend of the spine. If your chair has a straight back, you might want to use a small pillow or pad of firm foam rubber to support the lower back. Poor posture, from sitting in improperly designed chairs, can cause back problems, the second most common cause of visits to doctors' offices in this country.

If you don't have a good chair as described above, you should be particularly careful of the way you sit. You may have been taught to sit very erect with your buttocks pressed into the back of the chair, but in a straight-back chair this isn't too comfortable and it's a difficult posture to sustain over a number of hours. An easier way to sit in this kind of chair, and also more supportive of the lower back, is with the buttocks about three inches away from the seat back and the torso either slanted toward the shoulder rest (if you're talking or reading) or forward toward the desk (if you're typing or doing paperwork).

Another point about sitting which you may not know is that it is better for your legs and takes strain off your lower back if you have one foot higher than the other. When you lean over your desk, keep one foot flat on the floor and rest the heel of the other on the bottom portion of your chair. When you sit back in your seat, pull out a lower desk drawer and rest one foot on it. You might even keep a kick stool or small hassock next to your chair.

YOUR BODY IMAGE

Paying attention to the way you sit should make you more conscious of your posture in general. The way that you stand, walk, and move about your office says a great deal about you. You can't project an alert, self-confident image if you slouch and slump. Proper posture comes from having all parts of the body correctly balanced and in place. When one part is misaligned, your center of gravity is thrown off and some of your muscles have to strain to maintain equilibrium. This can be fatiguing.

To find your proper balance, start with your head. Move it around until you feel it balanced and equally weighted on your neck. Your head should feel light and loose, your neck elongated. Now examine your shoulders. If they feel tense and tight, relax them—but don't let them droop. They should hang easily and freely on the upper torso. Finally, lift your chest from the top of your rib cage. Stretching your upper body helps straighten your spine so it doesn't curve in an improperly aligned C.

Just as good posture helps you project a professional image, your body language when you sit in a meeting, walk into someone's office, or greet a client can work for you, if you're conscious of what you're doing. At a meeting, control nervous mannerisms like tapping your foot or drumming your fingers on the table. If you are nervous, and your hands are giving you away, find something to do with them or fold them in front of you. When you enter someone's office, walk in and take a chair rather than hanging back in the doorway. Finally, when you're introduced to someone, offer a firm handshake, not limp fingers.

DESK EXERCISES

If you need some bodywork—and who doesn't?—you can sneak some in on the job, even if you don't have the privacy of your own office. The following desk exercises will help your figure and relieve tension that may build up during the day. Jot them down on note cards and do a couple in between tasks or during your coffee break. They can be done pretty inconspicuously since they only take a couple of seconds each. Try them and see.

FOR STOMACH. Sitting up straight with feet flat on floor, push your stomach out as far as you can while exhaling deeply. Now inhale and pull stomach in tight. Do often during the day, holding the tucked-in position as long as you can.

FOR UPPER ARMS, BUST. Press palms together in front of you at chest height with elbows lifted. Push palms together as hard as you can, then release. Repeat a few times. Next clasp hands in front of you with arms in the same position as for the previous exercise. Locking fingers, pull your hands in opposite directions.

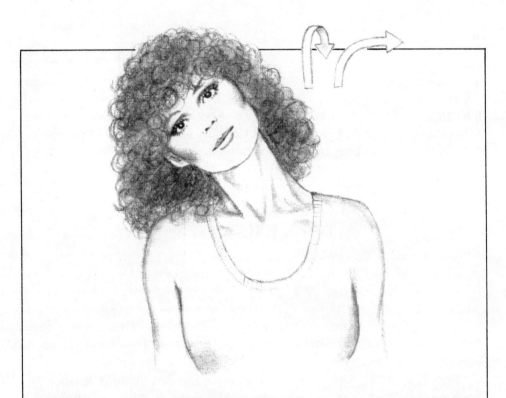

FOR NECK AND UPPER BACK. Drop your head forward, tucking your chin into your neck. Rotate head toward right shoulder, trying to touch your ear to your shoulder. Rotate head back, feeling the stretch in your neck, then toward left shoulder, again trying to touch your ear. When doing these head circles, keep the movement fluid and your shoulders relaxed. Do a few times in one direction, then reverse. Another exercise is to reach your right hand over your right shoulder, trying to touch the middle of your back. Bend your left arm behind

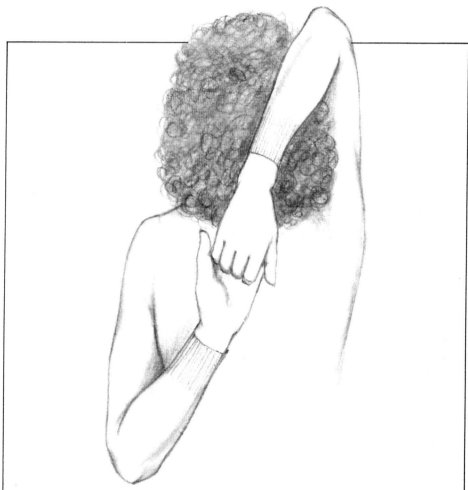

your back, and clasp your right hand. Locking your fingers, pull your
hands in opposite directions. Switch sides and repeat.

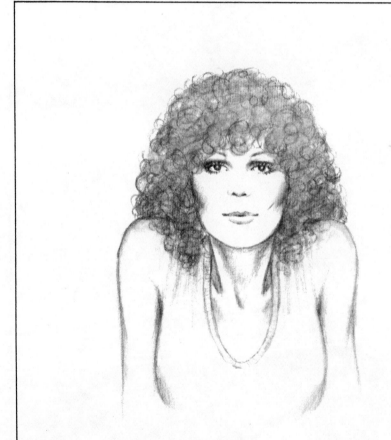

FOR SHOULDERS. Hunch your shoulders up by your ears, then pull them down as far as possible. Repeat a few times. Circle right

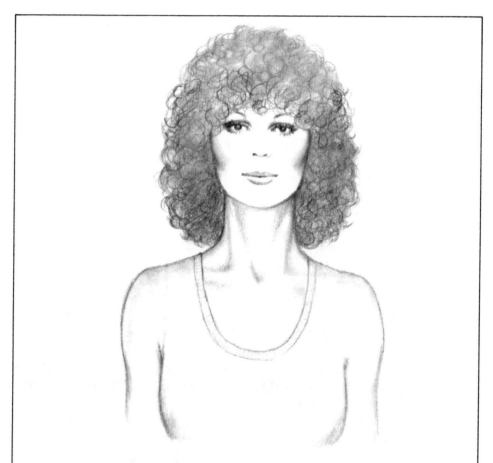

shoulder in a forward direction, then back. Circle left shoulder the same way, then do both shoulders together.

FOR PELVIC FLOOR. This is an invaluable exercise for preventing many "female" problems and should be done by every woman. Contract the muscles of your pelvic floor (the area between your urethra and rectum) hard for a second and then release. Repeat 10 times in a row to make up one set of the exercise (this takes about 20 seconds). In a month's time, try to work up to 20 sets in one day (about seven minutes total).

FOR FEET AND LEGS. Cross one leg over the other and rotate your foot in a circle. If you can, take your shoes off so you can really move your toes. Flex your toes at the top of the circle; point them at the bottom. Do in both directions with both feet. Also, keeping one foot flat on the floor with knee bent, straighten the other knee and lift foot off the floor. Holding this position, flex toes toward you, pushing heel away. Then try to curl toes over as though you're making a fist with your foot. Do a few times, then change legs.

If you have your own office or cubicle, your exercises can be a little more active. Instead of walking to the water fountain or coffee machine to reactivate your brain, try a couple of the following:

ARM CIRCLES AND CROSSES. With arms extended to the sides at shoulder height, describe small circles in the air, gradually increasing the diameter. Circle forward, then back. Next, with arms in the same position, swing them forward across your chest. Then swing them back as far as they will go. Repeat a few times.

ARM REACHES. Raise one arm above your head toward the ceiling. Look up and stretch as high as you can reach. Alternate arms.

FOOT SWINGS. Stand by your desk, with one hand lightly resting on the desk top. Swing one leg forward and back, keeping your upper body still. Repeat several times, then switch legs.

BEND-OVERS. Starting from a sitting position, exhale and lean forward till your chest touches the top of your thighs. Let your head hang over your knees, then inhale, and return to an upright position.
BODY PRESS. Sit erect with arms against your sides, grasping your chair seat. Push down with your arms while you try to raise your torso slightly off the chair. (This may take a little practice.) You can also try this exercise with your legs extended off the floor in front of you.
WAIST TRIMMERS. Rest your fingers lightly on your shoulders with elbows at shoulder height. Twist torso as far to the left as you can, then to the right. If you do this exercise sitting down, be sure not to lift buttocks from the chair seat. Next, standing or sitting, clasp arms above your head. With elbows straight, pull as far to the right as you can, then to the left. Repeat a few times.

You can get in some "accidental" exercise, just by getting out of your chair whenever possible. Set up your office so you have to move to get things. Don't keep all your books and supplies within reach. Take your phone calls standing up. Avoid elevators if you can, but for safety's sake, use stairwells only if they are fairly well frequented. If you work in a large office building, always check access to other floors before using the stairs so you don't get trapped behind a locked door.

By taking a few minutes out from work to do some of the exercises and follow the other routines suggested in this chapter, you'll find yourself fresher, less fatigued, and able to accomplish more. Your days will go better, and you'll look and feel better, too.

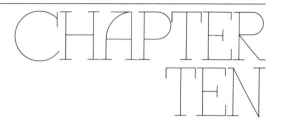

CHAPTER
TEN

Handling Lunch Hour With a Minimum of Calories

The hands on the clock are inching toward 12, and your stomach is telling you it's time to restoke. But what should you eat? When, where, and how? The answers to these questions will determine whether your lunch hour leaves you feeling refreshed and reenergized or depressed and sluggish. How you handle your lunch hour will also determine whether you stay slim and trim or slide toward "secretaria spread" and a widening waistline.

Whether you enjoy an expense-account lunch at the plushest restaurant in town or brown-bag it at your desk, it pays to be conscious of calories *and* nutrition. Sound, low-calorie meals will help you look better and feel better, and knowing that is an important part of any working woman's overall beauty strategy.

You can skip lunch to lose weight, as some women do, but you'll probably end up paying for it three hours later when you find yourself grabbing a 200-caorie candy bar to get you through the rest of the day. It is a much better idea to eat a well-balanced meal that will fill you and refuel you. By giving lunchtime some advance thought and planning,

Working
Woman's
Beauty
Book

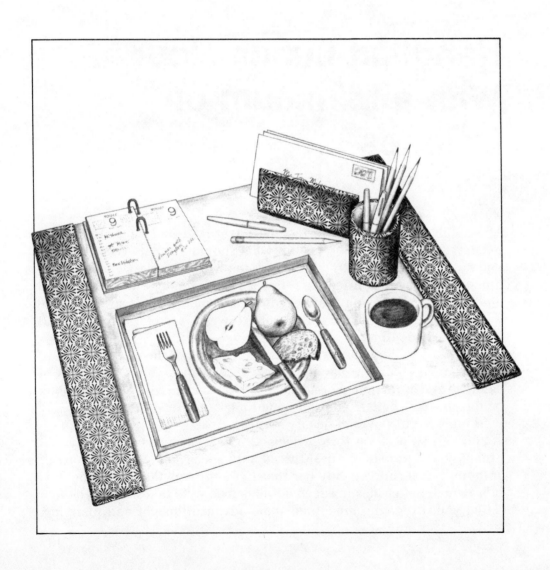

Handling lunch hour
with a minimum
of calories

you can do this without going overboard on calories. Here are some suggestions to cover a variety of situations.

THE BUSINESS LUNCH

The businesswoman's expense-account lunch needn't be the three-martini affair for which businessmen are notorious. If you want to hold on to your figure, and be able to get some work done the rest of the day save your drinking till after-office hours. This doesn't mean you have to act like Carrie Nation when the waiter asks if you would like a drink. If you are the one doing the entertaining, first ask your client or customer if he would like something. If he says yes, join him—but choose one of the following:

Virgin Mary: a Bloody Mary with everything except the liquor.
Spritzer: white wine and club soda over ice with a twist of lemon.
Lillet (pronounce lill-*lay*): a premixed dry white wine and seltzer with a splash of lemon or orange juice.
Kir (pronounce *keer*): white wine with a dash of Cassis (black currant liqueur) over ice with a twist.

If you want to be very chic and very sober, order Perrier (*pehr-ree-ay*) with ice and a slice of lime. This, according to author Michael Korda, the guru of status and power, is *the* in drink at places like "21" and the Four Seasons. The happy bonus is that it's good for you. A naturally carbonated mineral water that bubbles up from an underground spring in southern France, Perrier contains no calories, no additives, no artificial flavorings, or sweeteners. It is also high in calcium and virtually free of sodium for those on a low-salt diet.

Naturally, there will be occasions when you want to order wine with your meal, and a good businesswoman should be able to handle this capably. After the waiter has arrved with the menu, ask either him or the captain (if there is one) for a wine list. If you don't see anything you're familiar with on the list, it might be a good idea to pick a less expensive bottle. Moderately priced wine is more reliable; more expensive varieties must be drunk at the right age to be enjoyed to their fullest. There is no stigma in asking the captain for his recommendation, but if you feel funny about it, simply select a wine in the same price range as the entrée you've ordered.

As to that entrée, keep it as light as possible. Pass up casseroles and sauced dishes in favor of meat or fish, boiled or broiled. If you can't resist a roll while you're waiting, then forgo potatoes with your meal. Better yet, order a salad bowl, either with a squeeze of lemon juice or with the dressing on the side so you can control the amount that's put on. Try to skip first courses and dessert, but again, keep your guests company. If they order fettuccine, have some consommé or melon. Don't drool over their pecan pie and whipped cream; eat some fruit or cheese.

If you are acting as hostess, you should be the one to choose the restaurant. Keep in mind that French or Italian places abound in high-calorie temptations. A seafood restaurant or a place known for its

Handling lunch hour
with a minimum
of calories

steaks or grilled meats would be better. Chinese or Japanese restaurants are also good choices, and it's not a bad idea to spend a free lunch hour scouting establishments and window-shopping menus.

Once you find a place or two you like, stick with them. For a businesswoman, in particular, it is a good idea to establish a "home turf," where you are known to the management and help. For one thing, you will then avoid the hassles over bad tables or bad service that sometimes plague women, particularly when dining without men. Secondly, you can make advance arrangements with the maître d' to pay on the way out or be billed. That way, when you entertain a male client, you don't have to worry about wrestling for the tab.

To make sure you continue to get good service, don't be a stingy tipper. The standard rate is 15 percent on your before-tax food total, plus a lesser percentage on your bar bill. However, if you've become a fairly regular customer, you might want to leave 20 percent. This is easily figured by dropping the last digit from the pretax figure and doubling that amount. Of course, you only tip generously when satisfied with the service. If you're not, say something about it. That goes for the food, too. In order to carry off a business lunch as though you've been doing it for years, you need to be assertive about your likes and dislikes.

Having got through you meal with grace and style, don't blow your image by pulling out a lipstick or hairbrush at the table. Order your tea or coffee, then retreat to the powder room for a quick makeup check and to be sure you don't have a piece of spinach stuck between your teeth.

BROWN-BAGGING IT

At the opposite end of the spectrum from the luxury and leisure of the expense-account lunch is the quickie meal you eat at your desk when you don't have time to get away. But even when you brown-bag it or order from the corner deli, you can still make choices that are nutritious, filling, and easy on the calories.

When you have lunch sent up from the deli, stay away from egg, chicken, and tuna salad sandwiches, which are usually loaded with mayonnaise at 100 calories per tablespoon. Stick with sliced chicken, turkey, or roast beef, and only eat one side of the bread or roll. Live it up with the dill pickle spears, which are only three calories each.

If there is a grocery near your office, you can always hunt up small cans of salmon or tuna (packed in water, not oil), as well as containers of cottage cheese and yogurt. These last two items should not be considered meals in themselves, however, nor are they as dietetic as you might think. Creamed cottage cheese is 120 calories per half cup. The problem is that often the smallest containers sold are the one-cup size, which adds up to more calories than a plain hamburger. Yogurt is a great food, but if that's all you eat for lunch you should add a sprinkling of bran, wheat germ, or granola or mix in some fresh fruit to make a more balanced meal. Buy plain yogurt or flavors like lemon, vanilla, or coffee. The fruit preserves in the store-bought fruit yogurt add more than 100 calories and no extra nutrition.

If you bring your lunch from home, you have a wider range of choices and more control over the calorie count. Try these suggestions for a week's worth of brown-bag lunches.

Handling lunch hour
with a minimum
of calories

MONDAY
Fresh vegetable sticks
Hard-boiled egg
Lemon yogurt

TUESDAY
Cheese wedges
Slice of pumpernickel
Apple

WEDNESDAY
Cold roast chicken
Cherry tomatoes
Peaches

THURSDAY
Gazpacho
Saltines
Grapes

FRIDAY
Shrimp cocktail
Melba toast
Celery sticks

MONDAY MENU

Preparation: The night before, simmer egg(s) for 15 to 20 minutes while you peel and slice vegetables. Pack vegetable sticks over ice with a sprinkling of salt, and store in covered containers in the refrigerator to keep them extra crisp. The next morning, wrap sticks individually in small plastic bags. Stick the yogurt in the freezer overnight: it will be cold and slushy when you get ready to eat it the next day.

Calorie count: One medium carrot, sliced, 21 calories; one average cucumber, 29 calories; radishes are about a calorie each; and a ring of green pepper has negligible calories. Hard-boiled egg, 75 calories. Dannon lemon yogurt, 200 calories per container.

TUESDAY MENU

Preparation: Nothing to it (this is a good one for mornings when you're really rushed). Wrap cheeses in individual foil packets, the bread in foil or plastic. Grab your apple and away you go!

Calorie count: Choose 2 ounces of any hard, natural cheese; for example, Swiss, 88 calories per ounce; blue or Roquefort, 95 calories per ounce; provolone, 95 calories per ounce. Slice of pumpernickel, 74 calories. Small apple, 58 calories.

WEDNESDAY MENU

Preparation: Roast chicken in advance. Sprinkle chicken inside and out with coarse salt; rub with cut garlic clove. Then sprinkle inside and out with juice from one lemon. Roast one hour at 400°. Let cool, then cut and refrigerate individually wrapped pieces. Put small can of dietetic peaches in freezer overnight, so they will stay cold till you're ready to eat the next day.

Calorie count: Four ounces of roast chicken, approximately 200 calories. Cherry tomatoes (three or four small), approximately 25 calories. Small can of dietetic peaches, 80 calories.

THURSDAY MENU

Preparation: Mix gazpacho in blender the night before. Chop finely one tomato, half a green pepper, half a cucumber, half a small onion (use any leftovers from Monday's lunch preparation). Combine with 2 teaspoons olive oil, 1 tablespoon wine vinegar, 1 cup tomato juice, salt and pepper, a dash of Tabasco, and half a crushed garlic clove. Whir in blender about 15 seconds. (This recipe can be doubled, if you're feeding a family.) Chill soup and thermal container in refrigerator overnight. Pour in the next day.

Calorie count: Gazpacho, about 130 calories per cup. Four saltine crackers, 50 calories. Half a cup of grapes, 33 calories.

FRIDAY MENU

Preparation: Another quickie! The night before, place 4-ounce jar of shrimp cocktail in the freezer. It will thaw in about three hours the next day. Slice celery and pack with salt over ice until morning, then wrap in plastic bag.

Calorie count: One jar of shrimp cocktail, 110 calories. Melba toast, 30 calories per slice. Celery sticks, 6 calories per average stalk.

If you pack lunches for husband and/or kids, save time by preparing big batches of sandwiches and freezing. They'll keep two weeks or longer and will defrost and be ready to eat by noontime. Makings that freeze well are sliced meat and poultry, sliced natural cheeses like Muenster, Cheddar, and Swiss, tuna and salmon salads, peanut butter, and nut spreads. Do not freeze vegetables that you plan to eat raw as they lose crispness and texture. For more useful tips, write for a pamphlet called "Safe Brown-Bag Lunches." You can get it free from the Animal and Plant Health Inspection Service, Department of Agriculture, Washington, D.C. 20250.

If you eat at your desk regularly, you may want to keep the following on hand:

1. Silverware. A knife, spoon, and fork from home are more aesthetic than plastic utensils. You can rinse them off in the ladies' room.

2. Small plastic tray. Hunt up one about the size used to serve meals on airlines. By eating on this, you'll protect your work from spills and avoid having to explain coffee rings on your contract or report.

3. Dinner-size napkins. Keep a supply of these. They're more protection for your lap than the skimpy version the deli sends along (when they remember).

4. Immersion cup heater or electric hot pot. Handy for making coffee, tea, or instant soup. A four-cup pot that turns off automatically costs about $11.

5. Munchies. For mid-morning or mid-afternoon emergency snacks, keep small boxes of raisins, unsalted nuts, sunflower or pumpkin

Handling lunch hour
with a minimum
of calories

seeds. Or keep a small basket of fresh fruit (bananas, apples, pears) within reach.

At home, have on hand small plastic bags, a squat insulated thermos bottle, plastic containers with lids in a variety of sizes, and a zippered, lined bag to carry your lunch in. These bags come in lots of sizes and shapes at most notions counters. You don't want any disasters with leaking liquids in your briefcase.

CAFETERIAS AND COFFEE SHOPS

It's easy to get an overload of calories eating in the company cafeteria or the corner coffee shop. With cafeteria food you run into the obvious pitfalls of hot plates involving gravy and sauces, but you won't necessarily do better by choosing a fruit salad platter. If the fruit is canned instead of fresh, it has undoubtedly been packed in heavy syrup, and that in addition to a big scoop of cottage cheese can be pretty fattening. Try to stick with green salads (easy on the dressing), fresh fruit, a small wedge of hard cheese.

Similarly, don't fall for the "diet special" many coffee shops offer of a 3-ounce hamburger (minus the roll), cottage cheese, and jello. That can actually add up to more calories than you would consume eating a hamburger with one side of the bun, lettuce, and tomato (a half cup cottage cheese, 120 calories; half a hamburger bun, 60 calories). Better diet choices would be a cup of minestrone (or any soup that doesn't have a cream base), a two-egg omelet (plain or cheese), or a cheese sandwich.

To help you decide what is fattening and what isn't, you might want to carry around a pocket calorie counter. *The Barbara Kraus 1977 Calorie Guide to Brand Names and Basic Foods* (Signet, $1.25) is helpful, as is a chart called "Calories and Weights," which comes folded like a road map. The latter includes illustrations of actual serving sizes of meats to help you judge calorie values. It's available for $2.95 from Roy G. Scarfo, Inc., P.O. Box 217, Thorndale, Pa. 19372.

FAST FOOD

Now and then, everyone succumbs to the lure of the Golden Arches or "finger-lickin'-good" chicken. Fast-food eating needn't be junk-food eating, if you keep the following in mind:

○ Shakes and fries do little for you nutritionally and add more than 500 calories to a meal. Skip them.

○ When ordering a hamburger or a fish sandwich, "have it your way"—without the mayonnaise-based special sauces. Also go easy on the catsup (21 calories per tablespoon). Mustard (only 10 calories) is your best choice.

○ Having your burger or fish with a cheese slice adds 100 calories, but it does offer you protein, vitamin A, and calcium.

○ Eat only half of the bun and you'll save 60 calories. The top half with the sesame seeds has the most nutrients.

○ If you must have fried chicken, remove the crispy, and fattening, coating. Have a little coleslaw (⅔ cup, 68 calories), but pass up the rolls, potatoes, and gravy.

Handling lunch hour
with a minimum
of calories

◦ Pizza can be a good fast-food choice, so long as you don't load it up with pepperoni, sausage, etc. Stick to a plain cheese slice (regular, not Sicilian), and you will be getting protein, plus vitamins A and C, in just 155 calories.

◦ When you buy a hot dog from the street vendor, it's OK to load up on the sauerkraut; there are only 21 calories in a half cup. Just don't eat half of your roll.

No matter what or where you eat, try whenever possible to get in a little exercise before your meal. A brisk 10-minute walk before lunch will burn some calories and for some people acts as an appetite suppressant. Try it and see.

Vary your lunchtime routine so that you're not always eating the same food in the same place. When the weather is warm, eat outdoors; the change of scenery will be refreshing, and you can catch a little sun. Find a sidewalk café or take a picnic lunch to a park or zoo.

There are lots of things you can do on your lunch hour besides eat. You can visit the library, see a museum exhibit, take in a free concert or a short film. Check your newspaper for notices of special events. If you live close enough, you can even go home to walk the dog or take a quick nap. Lunch hour is also a good time to get in some exercise. Various kinds of workouts are described in the next chapter. Just remember that you shouldn't exercise right after eating. Go to your gym or dance class first, then eat something light on your way back to the office or at your desk.

CHAPTER ELEVEN

Feeling Fit

All work and no play make Jill a dull girl. It can also make her tired, tense, and possibly overweight. Riding to the office, taking elevators, and sitting behind a desk all day don't do much to keep you in shape, and poor physical condition can lead to flabbiness and fatigue. Studies have shown that lack of exercise can even make you prone to colds, allergies, backaches, and stomach problems.

Women have traditionally been relegated to jobs that do not give them a physical workout or require that they be in shape. A secretary, for example, uses only 78 calories per hour typing on a manual typewriter as compared to the 420 calories burned up by a coal miner. So physical fitness is even more important for those with sedentary occupations than for those with active ones. Richard O. Keelor of the President's Council on Physical Fitness and Sports considers the office desk and swivel chair "two of the most serious occupational health hazards" facing Americans today.

Ever since an experimental exercise program conducted by the National Aeronautics and Space Administration resulted in less stress and absenteeism and greater stamina among those office workers who participated, more and more companies have started setting up similar programs for their employees. They've got the message that fitness makes good business sense. You should get the message, too.

Of course, there are lots of personal benefits to be gained from a regular exercise program, among them improved strength, grace, coor-

dination, flexibility, and agility. While it has not been conclusively
proved that consistent exercise can prolong life or ward off heart
attacks, it is generally agreed that exercise promotes overall good
health and a sense of well-being.

Exercise has special benefits for women. The female body has a
tendency to store extra fatty tissue in the buttocks, thighs, and upper
arms. You may bulge in the wrong places—even though you are within
the limits on the standard weight-to-height charts—because your body
is high in fat. Only exercise will improve this condition. A regular
activity routine will help you lose inches, because toned muscles take
up less space than flabby tissue. And you needn't worry about develop-
ing the physique of Arnold Schwartzenegger. Even if you work out
strenuously, female hormones prevent women from building up huge,
bulging muscles like men's.

If you need to lose pounds as well as inches, regular exercise can do
the trick. The common myth that it increases appetite and leads to more
food intake has been dispelled. Dr. Jean Mayer, the noted nutritionist
who is now president of Tufts University, has demonstrated in carefully controlled experiments that moderate amounts of exercise actually suppress appetite slightly. Besides, lack of physical exercise, rather
than eating too much, is more often the cause of overweight.

In a recent study, Dr. Grant Gwinup of the University of California at
Irvine put 11 women, who ranged from 10 to 60 percent overweight, on
a yearlong program of walking, instructing them to make no attempt to
diet. (Each woman in the group had tried repeatedly without success
to lose weight by dieting.) No weight was lost until the women began to
walk more than 30 minutes a day. From that point on, the weight
gradually began to come off, and by the end of the year all had lost

Handling lunch hour
with a minimum
of calories

between 10 and 38 pounds for an average loss of 22 pounds.

These striking results make an excellent case for walking to work or at least hiking to and from the commuter station. If you must drive a car to the office, consider parking it several blocks away.

Besides giving you a better figure, exercise can improve your ability to cope with emotional and physical stress, a definite plus in any working situation. When you are getting your exercise, your heartbeat doesn't increase as much during tension as it does when you are out of shape. And after stress situations, your heartbeat returns to normal more quickly.

Exercise can also make you more mentally alert. Increased activity causes more blood to circulate to your brain at a faster rate, acting as a stimulant. Says one fitness advocate who spends her lunch hours working out at a gym: "When I'm done, I feel like working again. It's like the day is starting all over."

Finally, with all this muscle toning and psyche toning, exercise can't help but give you a better self-image, making you feel more self-confident and self-controlled. What further encouragement do you need? Get out of that chair and get moving!

COMPANY-SPONSORED FITNESS PROGRAMS

Once you have decided that you will start exercising, the next questions are how, where, and when. If you are fortunate enough to work for a company that offers a comprehensive fitness program you may be able to do your shaping up on company time. Unlike the corporate bowling teams of yesterday, these new fitness programs are designed to involve all employees, not just company athletes. What's more, company-subsidized memberships in spas and health clubs, formerly considered a "perk" for executives, are in some cases being extended to all employees.

More than 300 companies employ full-time fitness directors, but even the smallest company can start a program with the help of a doctor or fitness expert and the use of existing local facilities, such as schools or Ys. If your company doesn't have a program, you might bring up the idea. More information can be obtained by writing the President's Council on Fitness and Sports, Department B, Washington, D.C. 20201.

The types of programs available vary from company to company. For example, Life of Georgia, an insurance company located in Atlanta, features a gym, sauna and rooftop track, which can be used throughout the workday. At General Foods technical center in Tarrytown, New York, and at Zebco, a fishing-tackle company in Tulsa, Oklahoma, employees huff and puff their way around a Parcourse—a Swiss-designed landscaped track that *Time* magazine calls "a hybrid of miniature golf and the stations of the cross." About one-and-one-half miles long, the track is divided into a number of stations and looks like an enormous game board. A signpost at each station describes an exercise—toe-touches at one, leg-stretches at another—and directions for moving on to the next space. If your company doesn't have a Parcourse, but you're interested, good news! Franchises are creeping eastward from California and can now be found in 65 U.S. cities.

Completing the Parcourse circuit requires no small effort. When undertaking this or any other exercise regime, it's advisable to check with a doctor before you begin. This is especially important if you are over 30 or if you have not exercised at all in the previous year. Also, if you are over 35, you should have a "stress test." This involves pedaling a stationary bike or jogging on a treadmill for several minutes while an electrocardiogram measures your body's ability to handle strenuous effort.

Another popular kind of company facility is the Cardio-Fitness Center. Since 1972, Dr. Jerome Zuckerman, who has a Ph.D. in exercise physiology, has set up dozens of such programs, through his Cardio-Fitness Systems, Inc., for companies like Exxon, Mobil Oil, Western Electric, AT & T, Time Inc., and SCM Corporation. Usually companies subsidize a good part of the cost of membership for employes over 35; those younger can also join, but they pay more.

The typical fitness lab is usually open from 7:30 A.M. to 7 P.M. All gym togs, except sneakers, are provided, and showers and a sauna are available. Exercise sessions usually last about 35 minutes and involve working out with rowing machines, weights, treadmills, stationary bicycles, and other gadgets.

After taking a series of preadmission tests, including a stress test, to uncover those who may present a risk, you receive an individual "prescription" telling how hard and fast you can and should exercise. For instance, you may start on the rowing machine at 35 strokes per minute, then move up to 50 as your stamina builds and your cardio-vascular system (the operation of your heart and blood vessels) becomes more efficient. The idea is to get your heart working at 70 to 85 percent of its maximum capacity, or what is called a workout heartbeat. To find your target level, you can subtract your age from 220 and take three-fourths of that number. This should be the number of times per minute your heart beats when you are involved in good but nonexerting aerobic exercise.

Aerobics, in case you're wondering, means literally "in the presence of air." In reference to exercising, the term is used to distinguish those training routines that force the cardiovascular system to work hard from less strenuous routines like yoga or isometrics. Aerobic exercises are rhythmic, vigorous activities, like running, jumping rope, cycling, swimming, and brisk walking. The latest twist is aerobic dancing.

When sustained at a certain rate over a period of time, aerobics raises your body temperature, increases your heartbeat and breathing rate, and makes you sweat. If that sounds less than appealing, consider these benefits: A 35-minute workout for even two days a week will, according to Dr. Zuckerman, reduce your blood pressure (especially in people who suffer from hypertension). It will help you feel better, sleep better, and look better. And all that should improve your disposition. Other experts maintain that three 20-minute sessions every other day are needed for overall fitness, and that four sessions a week are necessary if you want to reduce weight and trim body fat.

If all this rah-rah exercise bit makes you want to yawn and prop your feet up on the desk, alternatives do exist. You could, for instance, join or form a company sports team. For years, men have been getting together at lunch or after work to play softball or basketball against teams from other companies. Well, the time has come for women to forsake their role as sideline spectators. Coed softball leagues are popping up everyplace. In Alexandria, Virginia, six-foot Susan Sachs has integrated the Time-Life Books basketball team, becoming the first female ever to play in a 25-year-old men's league.

Of course, if you don't want to lick 'em or join 'em, you can always assemble a female foursome for some noontime squash or racquetball. The point is to have fun while you're burning up calories. Just remember that for exercise to be beneficial, it must be done on a regular basis, not just when the mood strikes.

One final note on corporate fitness. You would do well to find out how your company's chief executive feels about the subject. Jogger Jesse Bell, president of Bonne Bell, was so interested in promoting running that he built a track near his Cleveland factory and paid employes $1 a mile to paddle around it, until some began lapping at $250 or more a month. Publisher Malcolm Forbes, who installed a physical fitness center at *Forbes* magazine offices several years ago, recently sent a memo to department heads letting them know what percentage of their people were using the gym. "Needless to say, I think exercise is incredibly important," says he.

If your boss has a similar attitude, it might be smart corporate politics to be seen working up a good sweat. And don't worry about it being considered unladylike. You're not a dainty sit-at-home type, but an employee interested in taking care of her body and health. Right?

PRIVATE HEALTH CLUBS

If you are so out of shape you don't want anybody you work with to see you in a T shirt and shorts, maybe it would be best to look for a private health club. Membership fees, which are not cheap, generally include use of exercise equipment, sauna, and a pool. Special services like facials, pedicures, and massages may also be offered, but you will pay extra for them.

To find a club, ask friends who exercise for recommendations. Visit the facility and try to arrange a free trial membership or at least an extensive tour. It's a good idea to visit the club at the hour you plan to use it to see how crowded it is. Is the pool big enough? Enough showers? Everything clean? Enough personnel to properly supervise equipment? What kinds of equipment are available? Don't be impressed by an array of machines that are supposed to "take the weight off for you." Things like vibrator belts are of little real exercise value.

Don't rush into anything. Before you sign any contract, read all the fine print. Take time to figure out how often you will use the facilities and estimate the price per visit. You can usually save money by joining for a year or more, but take a short-term membership at first to make sure you like the place. Paying for services you don't end up using is no bargain. Check, too, to see how long the club has been in operation. Sometimes the swankest new facility can go bankrupt within a year, and your money goes down the drain with it.

EXERCISE CLASSES

If you only want to participate in an exercise class, you would do well to check out the YWCA or adult education programs at your local college or community center. While you will be forgoing the sauna and the ambience of the private health club, you will save a lot of money. Here is a rundown on the kind of courses you may choose from.

BODY CONDITIONING. These classes are designed to strengthen, stretch, and tone your muscles, and they can be invigorating. You may use slant boards, dumbbells, and medicine balls. Or you may just work out on mats on the floor.

YOGA. Yoga is the most passive form of exercise, but that doesn't mean it's ineffective. A mental as well as a physical discipline, it increases flexibility, firms your body, and relieves tension. Using the proper breathing technique is essential, and regular practitioners claim that yoga conditioning reduces colds and other respiratory problems.

MARTIAL ARTS. Karate, jujitsu, kung fu, tai-chi, or what-have-you—it's an exciting way for you to stay in shape. Since speed and accuracy of movement rather than strength is the key, it is especially appropriate for women. The bonus is that in the process you may learn to protect yourself. And you never know when that could come in handy.

BALLET. For more romantic types, ballet classes will teach you how to move with grace while shaping up your body. In a basic ballet workout you use more of your muscles than you do in jogging, and it is just as good for your cardiovascular system. Just be careful not to overstress at first: Turning the feet out too far can cause ankle problems; too many deep pliés can tear knee cartilage.

TAP DANCING. Thanks to *A Chorus Line* and the nostalgia craze of the past few years, tap dancing has made a comeback. If you tap till you huff and puff, you may receive some aerobic benefits, but mostly this is for fun, more of a psychological lift than a physical one. Have you ever seen a sad tap dancer?

JAZZ DANCING. This is movement exercise done to music, ranging from early jazz to modern top-40 hits. It is good for your torso, provides an outlet for tensions, helps you develop freedom of movement throughout your entire body. Of similar benefit is **Belly Dancing,** which also teaches muscular control.

SWIMMING

Perhaps you would like to get some exercise, but on your own time and at your own pace. Then swimming may be an ideal fitness program for you. Besides being one of the very best methods for overall body shaping, it burns up an impressive number of calories: 400 to 500 an hour if you are a serious swimmer. The main problem is finding a pool big enough for a suitable workout. Again, be sure to check the size of the pool at a health club before joining. Y membership is cheaper, or check facilities at local colleges, high schools, and community centers.

Exercising in water is easier than on dry land because of body buoyancy. Total immersion in water reduces gravity's pull on you by almost 90 percent and makes swimming especially attractive to people with joint or muscle problems. On the other hand, the resistance of the water against the body builds strength and muscle tone. And just being surrounded by water stimulates the body's circulatory system.

If you decide to take up swimming, think in terms of a slow endurance-type plan. Start by doing a few warm-up exercises beside the pool, or do several minutes of flutter-kicking holding on to the edge. Swim for 20 or 30 minutes, alternating one lap of a strenuous stroke with one lap of a relaxing one. Or alternate vigorous laps with a leisurely walk around the pool. When you finish your laps, take five minutes to cool down—more flutter-kicking or walking or some deep-breathing exercises.

RUNNING

Another do-it-yourself exercise, though one in which you may increasingly find yourself in a crowd, is running. With the rise in popularity of this activity, you probably know at least one recent convert who is eager to rhapsodize on the virtues of pounding your local track or sidewalk. There are a lot of benefits to running: it's free, good for your cardiovascular system, and you can do it virtually anytime and anywhere. You don't even need to be well coordinated. Kathryn Lance, author of *Running for Health and Beauty* (Bobbs-Merrill, $8.95), claims that one year's worth of running cured her smoking habit, cleared her skin, changed her body, and improved her disposition. Even one out of those four would do for some people.

Such benefits, however, do not come without costs. Running *hurts*, particularly at first. Says Betty Phillips, cochairman of the Women's Long Distance Running Committee in New York City: "It takes about two months to get over beginner's boredom and pain." Bone spurs, shin splints, knee miseries, and bruised heels are the runner's equivalent of tennis elbow. To avoid these hazards, take the following precautions:

1. Before you begin your running program, walk briskly for at least a week. Add one more week of walking for each five years you're over 25. If you're overweight, add a week for every extra five pounds.

2. Invest in good running shoes. Do not run in sneakers. Look for a flexible shoe with a layered sole and elevated heel. Make sure it has

heel and arch support. If you will be running on pavement, wear two pairs of socks.

3. Never run after eating. Wait at least two hours after a meal.

4. Run flat-footed, not on your toes or the balls of your feet. If any part of your foot strikes the ground first, it should be your heel.

5. Increase your mileage according to the "talk test": If you can't talk while you run, you're going too fast. Running long distances at a slow pace is better for your health than sprinting. And the number of calories you burn per mile is about the same, no matter what your speed.

6. Always warm up before you run and do some extra walking when you stop. You need a cool-down period.

For more information on running, look up your nearest Road Runners Club, or write to the National Jogging Association, 1910 K Street N.W., Room 202, Washington, D.C. 20006.

JUMPING ROPE

For you closet exercisers, those who prefer to work out away from the eyes of the world, jumping rope may be the perfect routine. According to Sidney Filson, a New York woman who teaches classes and has written a book on the subject, there is nothing you can spend less time on, yet get more results from. "It gets rid of the flab that hangs from many women's arms," says Filson. "It lifts the pectoral muscles, it's good for reduction of the hips, thighs, and buttocks, and it burns up calories."

Then, too, you don't have to reserve a court, buy special equipment, or wait for good weather. A jump rope can also be folded up and packed in a suitcase, so you never have any excuse not to use it. Filson recommends jumping at least 15 minutes a day and considers a half hour ideal. The best time is first thing in the morning to get your circulation started and to set your energy level for the entire day.

As any eight-year-old will attest, it doesn't take much to get the hang of jumping rope. Still, there are a few techniques worth following. You should jump just high enough to clear the floor and look straight ahead, not down at your feet. Land lightly on the balls of your feet, with knees slightly bent. You shouldn't be able to hear yourself jump, nor should anyone one floor below you. Make sure the rope is long enough so that you can keep your arms low and close to your sides; most of the swing action should come from the wrists. Jump in sneakers or running shoes, not bare feet or you'll catch your toes.

Start at two to five minutes a day and work up to 15 or more. Set a timer and don't quit till it goes off. If you must rest, do some bending and stretching so you will still be exercising for the allotted time.

Whatever exercise you choose to do, moderation and patience are the key words. Several weeks of graduated activity allows your body time to adjust to the new demands you have placed on it. Don't push too hard all at once or you'll end up getting sore and giving up. Always be sure to do five to 10 minutes of warm-ups before starting any exercise and at least 10 minutes of cool-downs when you stop, so your body has a chance to gear up, then get back to normal.

Pick an exercise program that is something you like doing and that is suited to your pocketbook, personality, and recreational opportunities. Exercise must become a way of life if you are going to be fit and supple. It is as essential to your health and well-being as diet and sleep, and should become as integral a part of the day as brushing your teeth.

CHAPTER TWELVE

Learning That
Time Is Money

Assuming you don't have all the money in the world to spend pampering yourself, how do you decide when to pay for professional beauty services and when a do-it-yourself job is in order? The answer depends to a great extent on how much free time you have and how patient and skillful you are when it comes to things like fixing your own hair or doing your nails. While it is possible for you to perform just about every service discussed in this chapter, sometimes it isn't worth the effort and inconvenience. Home permanents are smelly; leg waxing can be messy, and if you don't know what you're doing, painful. Since you probably don't have a lot of extra time to spend on face, hair, and body upkeep, it might be worthwhile to pay someone else to "do" you during your lunch hour.

Before you make an appointment for any beauty service, from a haircut to a pedicure, be sure you know exactly how much it will cost and approximately how long it will take. Also, find out ahead of time what is included. Do you get a styling when you have your hair colored? Is a makeup included with your facial?

Here is a rundown of professional beauty care—what's offered, how much it costs, and how much time is involved. Prices are based on the going rates in popular salons in major cities. If you live in the suburbs or country, you will undoubtedly pay less, but you may not be able to find a comparable range of services.

HAIRSTYLING

A terrific haircut is essential for a busy working woman. Even if it costs $25 or more, it is worth the expense if your hair turns out looking great and is easy to handle. You don't have time to fuss with your hair, and you won't have to if you get a really good cut in the first place.

But how do you find a scissors wielder who can work this magic for you? Ask friends, even strangers, for their recommendations. If you see a head of hair you like, don't be afraid to go up to the woman and say, "Excuse me, I just love your haircut. Would you mind if I ask where you got it done?" Then you can visit the shop and ask for a consultation with the stylist. While there, check out the clients and the kind of haircuts they're getting. If everything seems in order, make an appointment.

At top salons, there is a separate charge for each service: shampooing, conditioning, cutting, blow-dry, etc. To save time and money, you may want to wash and condition your hair at home the night before. Then just ask to have it wet for the cutting. But before this step, see the stylist so he (most are men) can see what your hair looks like dry. This will help him judge what is the right cut for you.

If the salon is a popular one, it is a good idea to call an hour before your appointment to see how your stylist's schedule is running. You may save yourself an hour's waiting time thumbing through old magazines. Speaking of magazines, it isn't a bad idea to bring along clippings of styles you like. Sometimes you may know what you want, but have a hard time getting the message across. Pictures will help.

If you don't have any specific ideas and are a trusting sort, you may want to rely on the stylist's judgment and let him do what he thinks best. But first ask him to tell you what he has in mind. Always keep an eye on what is happening; if too much is being cut or you're getting nervous for whatever reason, say so. This would seem to go without saying, but many women are intimidated by their hairdressers. Fearful of offending, they will smile bravely and say they love the cut, then burst into tears as soon as they walk out the door. Keep in mind that you are paying for a service and that *you* are the one who must be satisfied.

After the cut, you may be turned over to the stylist's assistant for the blow-dry. Again, if you are in a hurry or want to save money, you can skip this step and either blow out your own hair or sit under a dryer or heat lamp. If you choose to have your hair blown dry or curled, watch closely and ask for advice on how you should do it at home. Remember, you don't want anything that is too complicated and takes a lot of time. If you think you will have trouble, ask to try the technique in the salon while the stylist watches.

Once you find a person who does a good job with your hair, you should have it trimmed every six weeks to keep it in good shape. The easiest way to keep track of the time is to make your next appointment as you leave the salon.

If you are still in the shopping-around stage, you can sample different salons cheaply by checking about "practice nights." These are special sessions when stylists are brought up-to-date on the latest cuts. By volunteering your head, you can get a free haircut supervised by an expert. The only hitch is that you may not get to choose the style. Ask ahead of time if you will have a choice or be required to go along with whatever haircut is being offered that evening.

PERMS

Perhaps you feel your hair needs extra help, something beyond a good cut. You might consider getting one of the new permanents that "retexturize" hair—changing fine to full, straight to curly, or coarse to controlled. Unlike the harsh perms of yesteryear, these are so loaded with conditioners that they do a beautiful job on any hair type, even streaked or bleached hair, which were previously considered unsafe to perm.

The major differences in today's perms are the timing and the way hair is rolled, using regular rollers rather than thin rods for those who want a soft, uncurly look. The new Sensor Perm system being used in many salons across the country takes the guesswork out of trying to figure when a perm has "taken." It monitors and controls the processing automatically by means of a small electronic device that attaches to any professional hairdryer. The machine buzzes when the hair has received the exact amount of curl desired.

Getting a permanent in a first-rate salon can cost as much as $50, but you can sometimes take advantage of advertised "specials" and get a reduced rate or a haircut, styling, and conditioning thrown in for the regular price of the perm alone. You can also try a home permanent, but for a successful outcome you must be able to roll your hair very neatly and be careful in timing how long you leave the waving lotion on. It isn't impossible to do a good job at home; however, it is tricky. A good salon perm may seem expensive, but consider that it will last from three to six months. You may decide it is a worthwhile investment.

Some salons offer "semi-perms" for about half the cost of a regular permanent. Rather than having the entire head rolled, about 15 rods are used in a rather random pattern to produce a smooth, almost straight look, but with extra body.

Unless you work in a very avant-garde field, you should stay away from any extreme styles, no matter how in vogue they may be. You want to look like a serious professional woman, and a headful of Little Orphan Annie ringlets is not exactly compatible with that image.

HAIR COLORING

Despite reports from the National Cancer Institute (NCI) in late 1977 that six common hair-coloring ingredients are suspected of presenting a cancer hazard to users, there has been no fall-off in the hair-coloring business. It is estimated that 33 million women use one type of hair color or another.

The suspected hazards stem from the fact that chemicals in hair dyes can be absorbed into the body through the hair and scalp. This would only be a danger with permanent hair-coloring methods. Most rinses do not contain the allegedly harmful ingredients. And with streaking or highlighting methods, only bleach (which contains no dyestuffs) touches the scalp. If you want to use permanent coloring and are concerned about the NCI report, send 50¢ to the Environmental Defense Fund, 1525 18th Street NW, Washington, D.C. 20036, and they will mail you a booklet listing those products that contain the potentially dangerous chemicals and those products that do not.

Home-coloring products are becoming increasingly easy to use, but most do-it-yourself jobs don't look as subtle as those performed in a salon. Still, home-coloring products are just $3 to $6, compared with the $25 to $85 price tags attached to the salon processes.

Any drastic changes, like dark brown to blonde, are probably best handled by professionals. But before making such a switch, consider seriously whether your new hair color will match the color of your skin and eyebrows. It's OK to go blonde, but only if the final, overall effect will be a natural one. Keep in mind that bleaching the hair to a lighter shade requires constant upkeep to make sure the dark roots don't show. It is also harder on hair than tinting, which does not change your natural color by more than a shade or two.

Highlighting—that is, adding touches of pale or deep gold to your hair—is one of the most subtle and attractive coloring methods. Some different ways to do highlighting include streaking, sunbursting, or tortoise-shelling. Since each of these involves treating only some strands of hair, you can do a lot or a little highlighting, as you prefer. The plus to these techniques is that touch-ups are not a problem; usually, one every three months is adequate.

In case you didn't know, you can have your eyelashes as well as your hair tinted at a number of salons. The black dyestuff used is a vegetable product, so the process is considered problem free. Tinting takes only

10 to 15 minutes and lasts four to six weeks, saving you hours of applying mascara. It costs about $10.

NAIL CARE

As a working woman, your hands are always on display. Split, chipped, or stubby fingernails can undermine the well-groomed image you want to present. If your hands are submitted to a lot of wear and tear during the course of a busy day, you may need professional help to get them, and keep them, in shape.

Nail wrapping is a kind of first aid for nails that split at the side and are in danger of breaking off. Very fine fabric or thin tissue is applied to the nails, then trimmed, shaped, and glazed over. This holds the nail together until the breaking point has grown out. Wrapping can also be done as a preventive measure to protect weak nails from damage. In a salon, the procedure costs $15 to $25, including manicure. If you have the manual dexterity, you can do it yourself with one of several wrap and repair kits sold at cosmetics counters for $3 to $4.

Another kind of nail wrap, available only in salons, uses plastic sheeting rather than tissue or fabric. The advantage to this method is that nails only need maintenance every two months, compared with every other week for the traditional wraps.

If you want gracefully curved nails but can't seem to grow them, or if your hands would be perfect except for one fingernail, you can have **nail extensions** applied. Extensions can be used on long or short nails equally well and are attached to the tip of the natural nail using a harmless adhesive. Next, a light coat of acrylic and a special liquid are applied, then smoothed down to blend into the nail for a remarkably natural effect. Extensions are healthier than full-size artificial nails, because by only covering the tips, they allow the natural nail to "breathe." It costs about $40 (manicure included) to have extensions applied to all 10 fingers. You can have just one nail repaired at a prorated price.

You'll pay about $6 for a regular manicure—cleaning, shaping, and polishing nails—and you may feel it's worth the money if you want a bit of pampering or feel it will inspire you to start taking better care of your nails yourself. When you have your nails polished, choose clear rather than colored lacquer unless you are very conscientious and can repair chips as soon as they happen. By the way, a manicure takes about half an hour, so to save time have it done while you sit under the dryer or heat lamps at the hairdresser's or while your facial mask "sets" at the beauty salon.

If you want your feet looking as good as your hands, you can have a professional pedicure (usually including foot massage) in about an hour's time. Any special foot problems—corns, calluses, or ingrown toenails—should be properly treated by a podiatrist.

LEG WAXING

If you dislike frequent shaving or applying depilatories, you might try leg waxing. Though waxing requires an initial investment in time and money, you don't have to repeat the routine more often than every six weeks, and the regrowth is not stubbly. Prices vary from salon to salon, as do waxing techniques. You can pay $12 to $30 for full legs; $7 to $18 for half legs. Most salons use some kind of hot wax, which is applied to the area, then either peeled off or removed with strips of muslin. It takes half an hour to get your legs waxed from the knee down, one hour for the whole leg.

You can do your own wax job at home using kits sold in drug and department stores for $5.50 to $7.25. The kits contain cold wax in a jar or tube, spatulas, and stripping papers. Or you can buy prewaxed cotton strips, which are even easier to use. Nonprofessionals are better off sticking with cold rather than hot wax, as it is water soluble and safer. Professional wax jobs are supposed to be painless; your home method may not be if you have a hard time removing the wax. Be aware, too, that waxing sometimes causes swelling and irritation. Try a "patch test" first to see how it works for you.

ELECTROLYSIS

Stray hairs on the face can be removed by electrolysis, a painless hair removal method that is permanent when done properly. The catch is that it takes more than one session and can involve a lot of time and money to achieve the desired result. During electrolysis, a high-frequency current is passed through an extremely fine needle inserted into the hair follicle. If the needle has been inserted at just the right angle, this zaps the papilla (at the base of the follicle) and causes it to stop growing hair. Of course, even the best technician won't score 100 percent. Expect about 35 percent of the hairs removed by electrolysis to grow back. To get rid of those, you will need a second treatment. Repeated visits may be necessary for very strong or curly hairs or those with twisted follicles.

Then there's the problem of undergrowth, dormant hairs under the surface of the skin that will crop up from time to time and need to be destroyed. Having electrolysis done frequently, twice a week during the first month of treatment, helps weaken undergrowth. After that, go once every few weeks until all hairs have been destroyed. You should thoroughly check out any electrologist before you go for treatment. Your dermatologist or family doctor can probably supply you with the names of qualified people.

Home electrolysis devices with retractable needles are sold for about $20. But they require a good deal of skill and patience.

DEPILATRON

Depilatron is another hair-removal method—more expensive than electrolysis—that uses electrical current. The hair itself, rather than a needle, is the conductor. Hairs are pulled out by a special tweezer, and there is no irritation or pain. Since no needle is used, the skin is not pricked at all.

FACIALS

Most professional facials consist of three basic steps. The first is cleansing: Makeup is removed, and a slough-off mask is applied and massaged into the skin with the fingertips until it rolls off in flaky crumbs, taking dry outer cells and dirt with it. The skin is then examined, and such imperfections as blackheads are removed manually. In some salons the skin is gently steamed, and impurities are drawn off with small electrical appliances—facial vacuums, as it were. The second step is toning. The skin is either massaged with special preparations, or a pore-tightening mask is applied to the face and neck to stimulate blood circulation. The third step is moisturizing, with creams, lotions, or sprays, to make the skin softer and more supple.

After these treatments, you are usually turned over to a makeup expert who does your face and no doubt tries to sell you some of the salon's products. Facials have become a big business at private salons. A number of department stores are now adding facial rooms to their beauty areas.

The purpose of all this masking and massaging is to deep-clean the skin and give it a rosy glow. Yet there are people who actually look worse after a facial. If the treatments are done too vigorously, those with very sensitive skin sometimes end up with a blotched or broken-out complexion. Women who have facials regularly claim they help keep the skin in top condition and firm the neck and face. Dermatologists, on the other hand, generally feel that though facials may be good for the soul, they don't do that much for your skin. The treatments are fine, they say, if you have the money and want to pamper yourself. But you can do as well for your skin at home if you take the time. (See Chapter 14 for information on home facial products.)

Of course, the sybaritic benefits cannot be denied. A complete salon facial takes an hour to an hour and a half and proceeds at a leisurely pace so you can relax and enjoy the experience. Some find the process such a great unwinder that they fall asleep during the massage.

You can spend $18 to $50 on a facial, including makeup, depending on the prestige of the salon you visit. If you take advantage of special programs offered by many salons from time to time, you can get either a reduced rate or free products included in the regular price. Watch newspaper ads for notices, particularly in the middle of winter and early spring. Another good deal that is sometimes available at department stores is the "minifacial," an abbreviated version for about $12.

FACE PEELING

Another kind of treatment for the face that is offered in a number of salons is the facial peel. This is a more in-depth process than the superficial sloughing of dry skin that may be part of a regular facial. Face peeling is done with creams containing mild chemicals (like resorcinol or salicylic acid) or parts of various plants (pineapple extract or papaya) that have a drying effect. When applied in a series of visits, these cause some of the top layers of skin cells to peel off. During the course of treatments, the skin becomes red and flaky, rather like the appearance of a bad sunburn. Because the face is sensitive at this time, sun and extreme temperatures must be avoided.

Given these inconveniences, plus the $250 to $500 price tag, why do women (or men) have face peels? The answer is either to rejuvenate the skin or to clear up a problem complexion. The operator of a famous New York City salon that features cosmetic peeling claims it makes long-range improvements in skin elasticity, texture, and muscle tone. The new layer of skin that replaces the one sloughed off is supposed to be clear and smooth. And sometimes it is. The results achieved are proportional to the extent of the original problem. Since only the topmost layer of skin is affected, the best you can hope for is to get rid of surface blemishes or superficial lines around the mouth and eyes. If your problems are more serious or recurring, you would be better off seeing a dermatologist or plastic surgeon.

Medical practitioners have two methods to remove wrinkles, acne scars, pigment marks, and other more extreme complaints. They can do a chemical peel with strong acids (phenol or trichloroacetic acid) or use a technique called dermabrasion, where the top layers of skin are sanded off with an electric rotary appliance. Both methods go much deeper than the cosmetic peel and, needless to say, are not exactly painless (though a topical anesthetic is applied to numb the skin). If you need to have these treatments, you may have to take time off from work while your face heals. But if you are bothered by scars, pockmarks, or wrinkles that make you look much older than you are, you may be willing to undergo the process and pay the $200 to $1,000 fee. It can make a great difference in your appearance, and perhaps your life.

MAKEUPS

As mentioned previously in this chapter, a professional makeup is usually included in the price of a facial. But what if you just want the makeup? Then head for the cosmetics section of any large department store. Policies on makeup stylings vary from counter to counter: A few are absolutely free, some may require a $25 minimum purchase, others charge separately for the styling in addition to required purchases. Know what you are getting into ahead of time.

Spending money on a makeup styling is probably a good investment, since it should help you find out which products and colors are right for you. And since dollars spent for cosmetics or treatments are wasted unless you know how to use the products correctly, it is worth your time and money to learn how.

Some cosmetics companies, among them Helena Rubinstein, offer seminars on skin care and makeup conducted by their own specialists. The nominal admission charge can be applied toward a purchase from the company's line.

The difference between a personal styling and a class is that in the latter you do, while in the former you are done to. For a personal makeup styling to be of real benefit to you, be sure you have a mirror to watch what the stylist does. He or she should explain each step, and you should feel free to ask questions.

Classes are usually held in community or meeting rooms at department stores. You will find tables set up with individual mirrors, tissues, and cotton balls. A professional stylist will demonstrate each step— sometimes on a subject chosen from the audience—while you follow along. If the group is a large one, additional stylists will usually be on hand to offer advice on colors and application techniques. You will learn how to cleanse your face, how to moisturize, how to apply foundation, cheek color, and eye makeup. Check newspapers for advertisements of these seminars. They can really be helpful.

TIPPING

Who gets how much? That is the question that must be dealt with after you have been pampered and prettied. To help you decide, here are some guidelines based on services and prices at leading salons in big cities; if you live in smaller towns the prices and the amount you tip will be proportionately lower.

Hair stylist	15 to 20 percent of the cost of the cut (When your hair is cut by the salon owner, you are not expected to tip.)
Shampooer	50¢ to $1 (Add an additional 50¢ if you have a rinse or conditioner applied.)
Stylist's assistant	$1 to $2 (depending on how much work he/she did on your hair)
Colorist	15 to 20 percent of the cost of the coloring (The same for the person who perms or straightens your hair.)
Checkroom attendant	25¢ to 50¢
Person who brings you lunch or snack	25¢

For other services:
20 percent of the bill for a facial
$1 to $3 for a manicure (depending on whether repairs were made)
15 to 20 percent of the bill for waxing and pedicures
$2 to $8 for a makeup artist

You can slip tips into attendants' pockets or use the small envelopes some salons keep at the reception desk. Tuck the money inside, label the envelope clearly with your name and the attendant's name, and leave it with the cashier. Remember that the difference between a good tip and a bad one is only a few dollars. If you tip generously, you will usually find that when you need to, you can call the salon at the last minute and be fitted into the schedule.

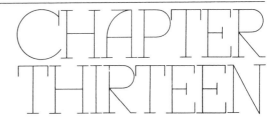

Making the Switch from Office to Out-On-the-Town

You're supposed to entertain a business client ... you have a dinner date ... a friend has tickets to the ballet ... it's the annual office party. Situations like these pose a difficult problem for the working woman: how to switch from your usual daytime look into a more glamorous evening one. Lynda Carter always seems to have a handy closet when she turns into Wonder Woman. Not only that, her transformation is accomplished in the blink of an eye. But how are lesser mortals to achieve an equally stunning effect without magic powers?

It isn't as tough as you may think. Using the suggestions offered in this chapter, you will be surprised at how much of a change you can make in yourself in just 15 minutes. You can disappear into the ladies' room or behind your closed office door and come out looking sensational.

WHAT TO WEAR

Many out-on-the-town occasions don't require too much of a change from your usual polished office look. There are several outfits that you can feel perfectly comfortable in by day that will still take you many places at night. Any of the following combinations has this versatility:

○ A skirted suit with a pretty blouse. Choose a classic suit fabric like wool or gabardine and wear it with a soft, feminine blouse. One with a high ruffled collar would be nice. Wear a handsome pair of pumps and carry a leather clutch bag, both in a dark color—wine or black, for instance.

○ A flowered challis dress. This go-everywhere look can be dressed up for evening with a pair of strappy, high-heeled sandals. You could also add a lacy shawl for a romantic touch.

○ A sweater dress. This is a wonderful solution during fall and winter months. You could choose a long-sleeved, cowl-necked version and add a metallic belt for evening. Or pick a sleeveless V-neck style with a matching cardigan. By day, wear the sweater buttoned over the dress. At night, take it off and toss it over your shoulders.

○ Dress and jacket. Another version of the sweater-dress-and-cardigan trick is to wear a soft, shirty jacket buttoned over a little nylon jersey dress—something in black with a bare neckline that you can uncover after office hours.

○ Skirt and blouse or sweater. Choose, for instance, a wool dirndl skirt in a smoky gray color. Top it with a silky long-sleeved blouse or soft sweater in white or a pale pastel shade.

○ Velvet blazer over pants. This is a perfect look for day that travels easily into evening. Wear with a stock-tie or drawstring blouse that you can loosen at the neckline for evening. The blazer and blouse can top a skirt equally well.

Of course, there will be occasions that call for a look that is too

Making the switch
from office
to out-on-the-town

dressy to get away with during the day. But you can still be glamorous with a minimum of hassle by simply switching one part of your daytime outfit, either the top or the bottom. For example, wear gabardine or velvet pants to the office with a sweater or cotton shirt. Change to a slinky halter or a glittery tube top for night. Or take a pair of crepe pants to the office in the morning to wear later with the silky blouse or tunic top that you paired with a skirt that day. Another bottom change: to a midi-length black polyester knit skirt (you can carry it to the office folded up, and it won't wrinkle). After you make your change, stick your daytime things in your desk drawer and tote them home the next day.

Accessories can be the key to dressing up a day look. For evening, add gold or silver bangles, some long chains or a crystal pendant and dangling earrings. Change your shoes and bag along with your jewelry. Gold, silver, or black patent leather are all dressy combinations. Finally, add a special evening touch: a silk flower, a black velvet choker, or a fringed shawl. The main thing with accessories is to limit the number of items you add and make sure they all work together. You don't want to end up looking like a Christmas tree.

YOUR EVENING MAKEUP

After a long day at work, you will probably want to clean your face to remove the day's smudges and oily buildup. Then, too, since your natural daytime makeup will be too colorless for evening, you might as well start fresh. To protect your clothes, you might want to tie a smock or apron around your neck while you do your beauty work. You could even keep a baby's bib on hand in a desk drawer. The plastic variety is useful because any spills can be easily wiped off. Pin back your hair with clips, don a terry turban, or stick in a few electric rollers if your set has gone droopy, and you're ready to start, with the supplies you've already stowed away in your desk (Chapter 9).

Step #1: Wash your face with a lotion, cream cleanser, or soap and water. If you use soap, bring your own from home. Institutional brands are too harsh for your skin. Remove eye makeup.

Step #2: Pat astringent (oily skin) or toner (dry skin) over face with a cotton pad.

Step #3: Dab on a thin film of moisturizer (dry skin) or blotting lotion (oily skin).

Step #4: Use wrinkle stick under your eyes and slick it over your lips.

Step #5: If you have dark circles under your eyes or an unexpected blemish, cover lightly with concealer.

Step #6: Apply foundation. Dot it on your face in several spots, then blend out evenly. Choose a shade from the suggested evening looks that follow.

Step #7: Pat or dust blusher on cheekbones, at temples, and under your chin to bring your face into focus for evening. For color selections, see the list of evening looks that follow.

Step #8: Apply lip color. You might want to use a brush to outline lips in a deeper color for dramatic effect. Choose a color to go with your total evening look as described below.

Making the switch
from office
to out-on-the-town

Step #9: Do eyes. First, make sure your lashes are clean and that your eye area is free from makeup remover. Dust your lashes and the area around the eye with powder. See suggestions that follow for eye makeup colors and shadow application tips. Carefully brush mascara on top and bottom lashes, wiping away any smudges with a cotton swab. Let mascara dry, then powder lashes again, and apply a second coat of mascara for thick, lush lashes. Make sure mascara is dry before using liner and shadow.

You'll want a couple of different evening makeups to use for different occasions and to go with different outfits. Here are three looks for you to choose from:

TAWNY AND EXOTIC

A rich and irresistible after-dark look.

Foundation: Use a warm shade one tone deeper than your usual foundation color.
Cheek Color: bronze or cognac
Lip Color: deep melon or wine
Eye Color: Use black mascara and a smoky wine-colored eyeliner. Starting at the midpoint of your eyebrow, streak plum shadow along the inner edge of your eye beside your nose. Use a deeper shade of plum on your lid, in the crease, and extending beyond the outer corner of your eye. Use a pink or heather highlighter on your brow bone.

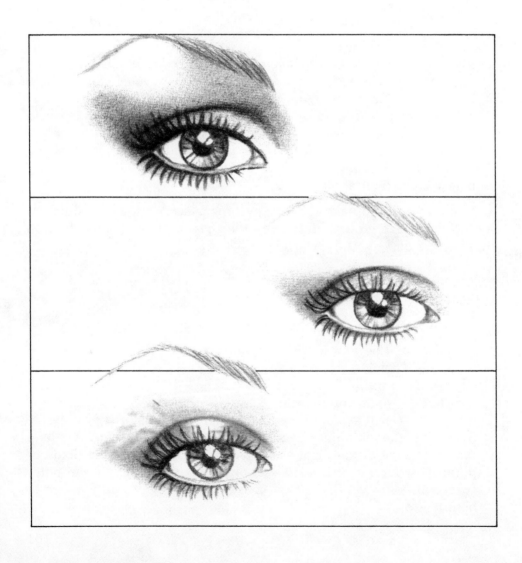

Making the switch
from office
to out-on-the-town

PALE AND OPALESCENT

A delicate, porcelain look that is both feminine and flattering.

Foundation: Use a cool shade in the lightest tone you can wear.
Cheek Color: cherry frost or red rose
Lip Color: shimmering pink or rose
Eye Color: Use black or brown mascara and a very fine rim of eyeliner in a charcoal gray or mahogany shade. Brush a dark blue pressed powder eyeshadow from the inner crease of your eye to the center of your lid, not extending above the crease. Then stroke a smoky slate shadow on the outer half of lid and gently smudge so there is no obvious line where the two colors meet. Use a powdered shadow in silvery sapphire to stroke on the outer edge of the brow bone; then wing it lightly in a semicircle to under lower lashes.

GOLDEN AND GLOWING

A shimmering, glittery look, great for special occasions.

Foundation: Use a beige-tone foundation.
Cheek Color: bronze or coppered coral
Lip Color: copper or a frosted gold shade
Eye Color: Use dark brown mascara and a mahogany eyeliner. For a gold-highlighted eye, cover your lid with a golden walnut shadow, then make a vertical line with solid gold pressed powder eyeshadow directly above pupils from crease of lid to lashes. Do not blend. To get the line centered, look straight ahead as you apply shadow. Dust a

bit more gold shadow on cheekbones and up along brow bone. For a final touch, wear a gold barrette in your hair.

With all the makeups above, blend colors well. When you get to your evening destination, check your makeup under the lighting there to pick up any mistakes.

WHAT TO DO WITH YOUR HAIR

One obvious solution to the what-do-I-do-with-my-hair problem is to go out at lunch hour and have it done. You can get a manicure at the same time, so your nails will be pretty, too. Unfortunately, there isn't always time for this treatment, so here are some easy do-it-yourself ideas.

   ○ Pull hair back from your forehead with a twisted silver cord for an updated version of those headbands you wore as a little girl. You could also use a thin velvet ribbon or a tortoiseshell band.
   ○ Fasten hair at the back of the neck with a silk flower or twist into a chignon.
   ○ Make an off-center topknot by pulling hair smoothly to the top of the head, slightly forward and just to the right or left. Fasten with a coated elastic, wind into a bun, and secure with hairpins.
   ○ Make a side ponytail by pulling hair behind one ear. Wrap a lock of hair around ponytail and insert a fan-shaped hair ornament.
   ○ Part hair down the center of head and use two combs to pull hair back and away from the temples. To insert a comb, pull it through

Making the switch
from office
to out-on-the-town

your hair, top side down, to spot you want to attach it. Flip comb so the right side faces up, then push it forward to secure.

    ○ Another variation is to pull hair back on one side with a comb and let the other side fall loosely. Use a sleek, sculptured comb in gold- or silver-tone metal, or a plastic one with a tortoiseshell bar.

AVOIDING HANGOVERS

If you're going out on a weeknight, you really can't afford a hangover the next day. Who needs a splitting headache, churning stomach, and furry tongue at the office? Before you head for a party or an evening out where there will be a lot of drinking, do yourself a favor and have a substantial protein snack. Bring from home or save from lunch a piece of cheese or a hard-boiled egg, or have a container of yogurt delivered to your desk at about 4:30. Not only will the food help line your stomach (so alcohol will be absorbed into your bloodstream more slowly), but a pre-party snack will suppress your appetite so you won't gobble too many fattening hors d'oeuvres.

As to what you drink during the evening, remember that the amount and kind of alcohol you consume will probably affect how you feel the next day. You might keep in mind the suggestions offered in the business lunch section. Wine is usually about 11 percent alcohol, compared with Scotch at 40 percent and vodka at 46 percent. If you consume mixed drinks, try to dilute them by adding extra ice. The traditional advice about not mixing liquors is also good to remember. Don't switch from cocktails to wine to liqueurs. Choose your drink and stay with it, if you want to keep a clear head. By pacing your drinks so that you take 30 to 45 minutes to finish one and continuing to eat while you drink, you should be able to get through even the longest evening fairly sober.

Naturally, there will be occasions when you want to celebrate and throw caution to the wind, and this is fine—provided you're not entertaining clients or don't have any major tasks ahead of you at the office the next day. But only "tie one on" when you feel relaxed and happy, not tired and tense. According to some experts, you are more likely to develop a hangover when you are emotionally depressed. If you decide to live it up, do so without remorse and you might not have to pay for it the next day.

BEFORE-BED ROUTINE

As tired as you may be when you get home, don't neglect to remove your makeup. Your skin needs to breathe and will be better off in the morning if you take care of it the night before. Waking up to old, smudgy makeup is no treat and is likely to bring out the worst in your complexion. Take a minute either to wash your face or tissue off makeup with cleanser. Use eye makeup remover, too, to get off all your mascara so you don't have a pair of black eyes in the A.M.

Since skin tends to be dehydrated by alcohol, late hours, and smoke-filled rooms, apply a thin film of moisturizer all over your face before you go to sleep. Avoid heavy creams, which can trap excess fluid that accumulates during the night and causes puffiness. Pat eye oil wrinkle

Making the switch
from office
to out-on-the-town

stick over any lines under your eyes, and slick it on your lips to keep them from feeling dry and parched in the morning.

You might also want to slip into a warm tub for just a few minutes. You may be tired physically, but wound up mentally from the evening. A short soak will relax and soothe you so you can drop off to sleep more readily.

Some people say that two aspirin before bed, even if you're feeling fine, will ensure a headache-free morning after. (If you're prone to upset stomachs, try the buffered variety or an aspirin substitute.) Others swear by a glass of milk to line the stomach, or several glasses of water to flush out the system. Dr. Seymour Diamond, author of a book on headache remedies, recommends a few teaspoons of honey on toast or crackers before bed. Honey contains fructose, a kind of sugar that helps your body to metabolize alcohol faster, thereby reducing the chance of a hangover, according to Dr. Diamond.

THE MORNING AFTER

No doubt you want to stay in bed, but force yourself up and into the shower. The spray will get your blood circulating and you'll feel more alive in minutes. To make it even more invigorating, give yourself a brisk rubdown with a loofah, a fibrous natural sponge. If you can squeeze in the time, shampoo your hair to get rid of lingering smoky odors and make you feel better later on. Nothing is more of a drag on your morale than to have to look at limp, stringy hair in the mirror all day.

If your skin needs a pickup, you could try a stimulating mask. The brush-on, peel-off kind takes only a few minutes and can revive tired skin and give it a healthy glow. If your skin is dehydrated, you might steam it by bending over a pot of hot chamomile tea for a few moments, with a towel over your head like a tent. If you don't have time for this, just lean over a sinkful of warm water and splash. Pat on moisturizer while your face is still a little wet to lock in extra moisture. Drink a couple of glasses of water, too, to replace fluid in your body tissues.

Walking, exercising, and drinking coffee are thought by some to be good remedies for a hangover. But forcing activity and stimulants on an already fatigued body can be like whipping a tired horse. Instead, try some yoga breathing. Sit cross-legged on the floor with eyes closed and arms resting lightly on knees. Breathe in slowly to a count of eight, then exhale to another count of eight. Push your stomach out as you exhale, pull it in as you inhale to take in as much air as possible. Repeat several times before getting dressed and putting on your makeup.

As to makeup, chances are you look tired and pale, but don't try to compensate by overdoing your makeup. Stick with clear, bright colors and use a light touch. Too much makeup will clog your skin and look like a mask. Dark colors will only emphasize weary eyes and call attention to pallor. A tip for puffy eyes: Rubbing them very lightly with an ice cube will reduce swelling, tighten pores, and help erase tiny lines. If eyes are bloodshot, use clear-up drops and wait a bit before applying mascara.

To perk up your color, wear a bright shirt or a cheery scarf around your neck. To pick up your spirits, buy a small bunch of flowers on your way to work to put in a vase on your desk.

CHAPTER FOURTEEN

Finding Ways
to Unwind

One of the main reasons women have tended to live longer than men is because until recently we have not been subject to the occupational hazards which accompany big-league, high-pressure jobs—that is, heart attacks and strokes. We haven't been privy to that level of decision-making for long, so we haven't had the worries that go along with it. The question that arises as women make strides into areas previously closed to us is this: If stress is a necessary by-product of most exciting and challenging jobs, how can we achieve success without paying too high a price for it?

The answer lies in mastering certain basic techniques for dealing with pressure. Many business schools now offer seminars that teach executives how to cope with stress, both their own and that of their employees, and a number of books have recently been written on the subject.

Authorities define stress as anything that places a demand on the body. That demand is referred to as a "stressor," and it can take almost any form: a job transfer, a traffic jam, a vending machine that doesn't work. Even good things, like receiving a promotion or going on vacation, are considered stressors.

If you stop and think about it, you can probably list dozens of sources of stress that you deal with on a day-to-day basis. For the most part, these do not cause you any great problems. Dr. Hans Selye, an expert on the subject, believes that each of us inherits a fixed amount of resistance to stress, which he calls "adaptation energy." It is when you expend too much of your adaptation energy that you may be headed for high blood pressure, migraines, ulcers, or other physical manifestations of stress.

Before things go that far, you would be wise to learn ways to release tension and reduce anxiety, and to incorporate these antistress practices into your daily routine. You may feel you can't take time to relax completely, but in fact you can't afford not to.

RELAXATION EXERCISES

One way to cope with stress is to be able to "let go" physically—to know how to drain tension from your body. One easy relaxation technique you can do right at the office whenever you feel yourself tightening up is to close your eyes and take several deep breaths, holding each one for a count of five and saying the word "relax" as you exhale. This may sound too simple, but it is a bona fide behavior-control mechanism that was developed through research. By repeating this procedure for one or two minutes, you can slow down your heart rate and neutralize, at least for the moment, the stimulus that is causing you to be uptight.

A variation on this theme is described by Dr. Herbert Benson in his best-seller *The Relaxation Response* (G.K. Hall, $9.95). To combat stress, Dr. Benson advises you to breathe through your nose, all the while repeating a single-syllable word such as "one" each time you exhale. He recommends continuing this pattern for 20 minutes at a time, letting your thoughts drift. If you practice this technique for long, you will find that its simplicity is deceptive. It takes a real effort of will to set your mind free from immediate problems. If you can train yourself to do it, however, you are likely to experience a surprising sense of inner peace.

To release tensions that result from sitting hunched over your desk all day—neck, back, and shoulder aches—you can use the exercises described in Chapter 9. The head rolls and shoulder lifts are particularly helpful. Another way to relax tense, knotted muscles is to sit in a chair with your eyes closed. Clench one of your fists as hard as you can. Then let your entire arm go limp. Do the same with your other fist and arm. Next, raise your eyebrows and crinkle your forehead. Then relax. Repeat this tense-relax pattern through all your body parts right down to your toes. When you finish, sit quietly for a few moments before opening your eyes.

REST POSTURES

After a long day of work, you need a proper rest period to reenergize your body. If you don't have time for a nap before fixing dinner or plunging into whatever you have planned for the evening, one of these postures should help refresh you and give you a new burst of energy. Try one for five to 10 minutes as soon as you get home from the office:

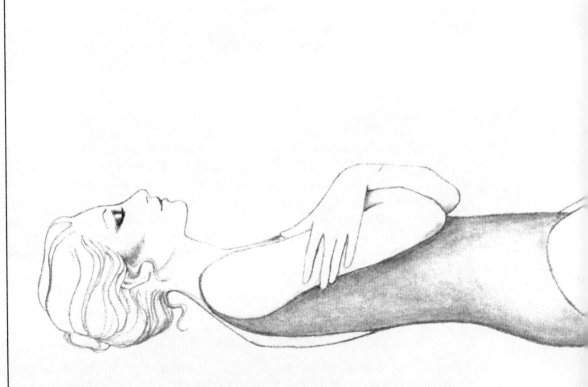

RAG DOLL. Lie on the floor with knees bent and two pillows underneath them for support. Crisscross your arms over your chest as if you were hugging yourself. Now imagine you are a rag doll with no

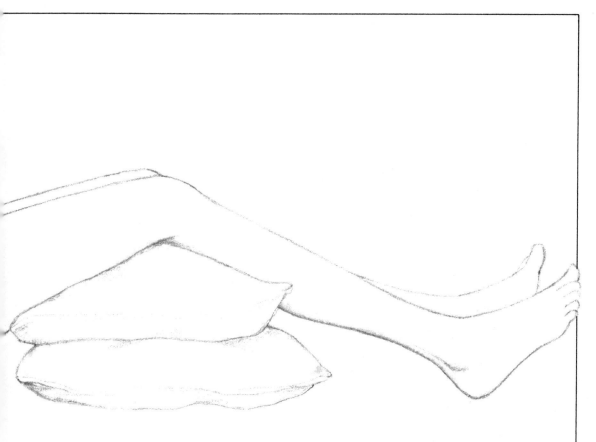

bones, no muscles, no joints. It ought to be easy if you are really tired. Close your eyes and let all your body weight sink into the floor. Breathe deeply.

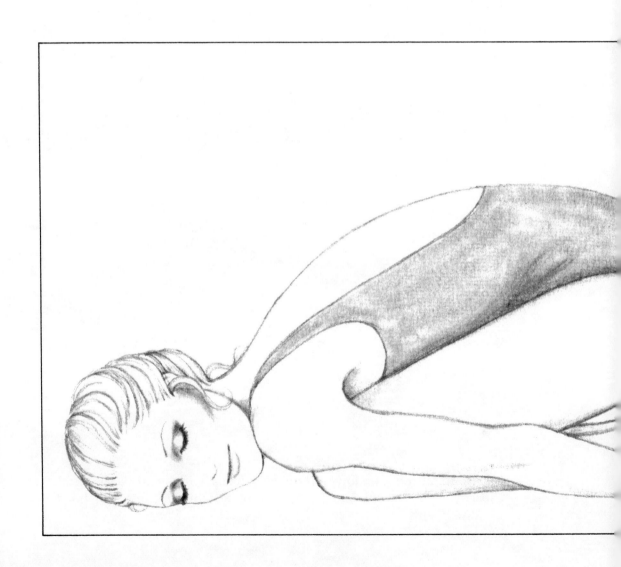

DYING SWAN. Kneel on the floor, then bend chest forward to touch the tops of your legs. Turn head so that one cheek is against the floor, and stretch arms out at your sides, palms up. Close your eyes and hold this position, relaxing all tension out of your back and shoulders and breathing deeply.

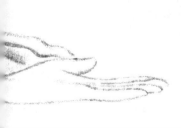

You can also lie down on your bed and elevate your legs by propping your feet up against the wall. The important thing with all these procedures is to keep your eyes closed and let your mind float. Don't retrace all the things that went wrong during the day. Make a conscious effort to clear your head of everything but tranquil thoughts.

Stretching exercises will also feel good after a tense day. Stand up and stretch your arms over your head as high as you can reach. Then drop arms down to the floor, bending your knees as you do. Hang there loose and limp, and then bounce gently for a count of 10. Straighten up and repeat.

You should stretch from a lying-down position as well. Get down on the floor with arms at your sides and legs relaxed. Raise arms above your head and reach out with fingers and toes, trying to elongate your body as much as possible. Return arms to your sides and relax legs, then repeat the stretching. Do several times. It is essential that you breathe properly as you do this exercise. Remember: Inhale when you stretch, exhale when you release.

While you're there on the floor, try the **pelvic tilt**: it's good for your back after a day of sitting. Lie down with knees bent and feet flat on the floor, chin tucked in against the neck. Put your fingertips under the small of your back, in the space where the spine arches slightly away from the floor. Now by tightening your abdominal muscles, press your lower back against your fingertips. You should be able to close up the space so that your back is pushing into the floor. Release slowly, then repeat several times.

THE SOOTHING SOAK

There is nothing like a leisurely bath to soak your anxieties away. After an especially harrowing day, you deserve a little private pampering. Even working mothers with young children should be able to grab at least 15 minutes alone. Put dinner in the oven, plunk the kids in front of *Sesame Street,* or let Daddy entertain them, and go lock yourself in the bathroom.

Fill your tub with warm water, not hot. It isn't true, though many people think so, that the hotter the bath the greater the relaxation. An extra hot bath steps up your metabolism, which forces the heart to work harder and will actually leave you feeling more fatigued afterward. If you desire a truly tranquilizing soak, the water temperature should be between 100° and 110°F.

To enhance the psychic and physiological benefits of your bath, add oil, bubbles, or salts. A milk bath softens the water as it cleanses, conditions, and perfumes the body. Run a little water in the tub, then sprinkle in the fragranced white powder. Turn the tap on hard to bubble up a rich, creamy, long-lasting foam.

Other accessories to make your bath more pleasant include

* an emollient, scented soap on a wristlet
* cleansing gel to squeeze on a sponge or apply directly with your palm
* an inflatable bath pillow
* a tub tray to hold a book and a glass of chilled wine
* a long-handled back brush for hard-to-reach spots
* a large natural sponge or a loofah, a dried sponge that looks like a long, flat scouring pad when you buy it. After a few minutes' soaking in water, the loofah plumps out and softens a bit. Used on your arms, legs, and back in place of a washcloth, it will polish away rough spots and allow your satiny natural skin to shine through.

While you're in the tub you can read or listen to soft music or just close your eyes and meditate. If you really want to go all out, light a few scented candles and turn off the bathroom light. It does wonders!

Something else you can do in the tub is exercise—nothing strenuous, of course, just a few stretches. But be sure you have a rubber mat under you so you don't slip. To stretch the backs of your legs, loop a washcloth around one foot and pull it gently toward you, keeping your knee straight. To limber your spine, reach high over your head while holding a washcloth tightly with two hands. Bend forward until you can pass the washcloth over your toes. To work on your pectoral muscles, hold arms straight out in front of you and squeeze a bath sponge between clasped hands. You can also do the foot flexes, shoulder hunches, and head circles described in Chapter 9, if you weren't able to fit them in earlier in your day.

If you are not the tub type, a shower still offers soothing possibilities. Turn the warm water on full blast and just lean into the pleasure. Wash your hair if you want to, but don't be in a hurry to get out. Stay under at least five minutes doing absolutely nothing. True sybarites might want to invest in one of the new shower heads that adjust to different sprays or pulsate to give a brisk shower massage. Some models come equipped with extra body and bath-brush attachments. The hand-held, or "telephone," shower attachment is practical for women because it can be aimed so you don't get your hair wet if you don't want to. Different models range from $20 to $100, and most can be installed fairly easily by removing the present shower head and screwing on the new one. Some special attachments require the assistance of a plumber.

Did you know that your bathing habits may provide a clue to your true nature? According to Dr. Ernest Dichter, founder of the Institute of

Motivational Research, people who prefer a shower tend to be more matter-of-fact about themselves and less self-indulgent than people who would rather soak in a tub. Those who expose themselves to the full force of a shower are more likely to face life head-on, says Dr. Dichter, while tub people are usually more self-protective and comfort loving.

Whether you choose tub or shower, an after-bath ritual can extend your period of relaxation. When you get out of the water, apply a lush moisturizer to add a silky gleam to your body while it softens and scents you. Let your fingers knead the lotion into your legs, arms, and shoulders. Or use a massage machine that spreads lotion on your skin via a rotating disk.

MASSAGE TECHNIQUES

A good massage can be marvelously relaxing and sometimes energizing as well. As such, it offers another way to cope with everyday stress. You can seek out the services of a professional masseuse or exchange rubdowns with a friend or member of your family. According to many teachers of the art of massage, the most effective ones are apt to be those exchanged by people who care about each other. A number of courses and workshops on massage have cropped up around the country, along with several books on the subject. You might check your local Y or continuing-education programs to see what is available in your area. There are several different massage techniques, among them the following:

SWEDISH MASSAGE. Vigorous kneading of muscles and drumming on flesh with long, firm strokes to get circulation going.

SHIATSU. Japanese massage accomplished by pressing down hard, mainly with the thumbs, on the body's acupuncture points. According to shiatsu theory, energy travels through the body along 12 meridians, and pressure applied to the *tsubas* (the acupuncture points along each meridian) takes care of blocked energy and gets it flowing evenly again.

REFLEXOLOGY. This type of massage treats internal disorders ranging from headaches to heart problems by manipulating particular areas of the feet. The theory is that each body part has a reflex point in the feet.

One of the valuable things about massage is that you can learn to recognize your own areas of bodily tension and find out how it feels to be truly relaxed. This will help you with the relaxation exercises described earlier in this chapter. Also, tuning in to your body can provide an emotional high—particularly if you have been so preoccupied with what was going on in your head that your body was disappearing from your experience.

When giving or receiving a massage, keep these pointers in mind:

1. You need a warm room for the proper setting and some body oil to reduce skin friction.

2. Beds are too soft to lie on for a massage, but a thin mattress, exercise pad, or sleeping bag placed on the floor will do fine.

3. A good massage is best accomplished in dim light and a peaceful atmosphere. Soft, slow background music is nice. The procedure should take about 20 minutes.

4. Though you'll need to read a book or take a course to understand the fine points of shiatsu or reflexology, Swedish massage requires very little preparation. Try these basic strokes:
* **Effleurage:** long, firm strokes, always toward the heart, using your palms or the balls of the fingers;
* **Pétrissage:** a kneading process, like kneading bread, wherein you lift up skin and muscles and roll them around between your fingers;
* **Friction:** small, hard circles on the skin, using thumbs or fingers around joints, palms for the back.
5. When you are the person giving the massage, lean into it with your whole body, not just your hands and fingers. But relaxation, not pain, is what you're after, so keep asking the other person how it feels.
6. Do each stroke at least twice and maintain light hand contact with the person you're massaging. Continuous skin-to-skin contact is essential.

RELIEVING HEADACHES WITH MASSAGE

Believe it or not, it is often possible to get rid of tension headaches by using a do-it-yourself massage technique. If you come home from work with your head throbbing, try this method recommended by Dr. John Upledger in his book *An Osteopathic Doctor's Treasury of Health Secrets* (Prentice-Hall, $8.95). Lie flat on your back on a firm surface without a pillow. Place your middle fingers in the groove between the base of your skull and your neck. Crooking your fingers, try to spread the muscles at the base of the skull in a sideways direction, going slowly and using the same pressure on both sides. This should relax the muscles of the upper neck and relieve much of the pressure that contributes to headaches. Keep rubbing until muscles seem looser to the touch. As the muscles relax and the groove deepens, your headache should diminish.

Dr. Upledger also claims that you can alleviate eye strain and secondary headaches by massaging specific areas for about 30 seconds daily. To find these spots, put your hands behind your head and feel around the back of the neck with your middle fingers till you find places that are tender when pressure is applied. These spots should be massaged gently but firmly, using circular motions.

HELP FOR TIRED FEET

As mentioned earlier, foot reflexology involves massaging points in the feet in order to relax various organs, muscles, and glands in the rest of the body. According to reflexologists, your big toes represent your head, the inside base of the big toes your throat, the arch your spine, the ball of the foot your thyroid, and so on. When a part of the body is congested with tension, its reflex point will be tender to the touch. Massaging the feet, reflexologists contend, helps facilitate natural healing processes and makes tender spots disappear.

Even if you don't go along with the sum total of this theory, you will likely find foot massage to be wonderfully relaxing. And because you can do it yourself, it is a handy technique to have in your bag of antistress tricks.

Before you massage your feet, soak them in warm, soapy water and use a good pumice or abrasive callus remover. Or you might try this routine: Fill a basin with hot water (as hot as you can stand, this time) and place it in the bathtub. Then turn on the cold tap. Alternately plunge your feet into the hot basin for a count of 10, then under the cold water for another 10 count. Repeat twice, then blot feet dry. For another quick pickup, you could use a facial mask on your feet.

After these procedures, massage feet with a rich cream or lotion. Apply a little bit at a time, rubbing it in by drawing hard little circles over the sole of your foot with the knuckles of your hand. Next, take your foot in your hands and make the same kind of circling motions with your thumbs, covering the sole and top of the foot.

Now hold your foot in both hands, with your fingertips meeting in the middle of the sole and the heels of your hands touching on top. Gripping hard, slide your hands apart very slowly. Repeat several times. Finally, take the big toe between your index finger and thumb. Twisting your fingers from side to side, gently pull until your fingers slide off the end of the toe. Do this with all your toes.

HELP FOR TIRED SKIN

Facial masks are a boon for perking up the skin and giving it a rested look after a tiring day. When you use a mask, choose a formulation right for your skin type. Dry skin, for example, needs creamy clay mask to tone, tighten, and brighten the skin without drying it out. Oily skin needs an astringent mineral mask to control excess oil and unclog and refine pores. Both help slough off dead, dry surface cells and leave the face with a finer finish.

Another popular mask is the brush-on, peel-off variety. A thin liquid film is spread evenly on the face and allowed to harden into a latex covering, which is peeled off in one piece. Because the mask shrinks as it dries, it gives the skin a temporary ironing and stimulates circulation to provide a pleasant glow.

If you have very dry skin that often looks lined and worn, you might want to try a petroleum jelly heat pack. Clip your hair out of the way, cleanse your face thoroughly, and then cover it with petroleum jelly. Dip a small towel in hot water and wring it out well. Then lie back in a reclining chair or in a bed propped up by pillows and cover your face with the hot towel for 15 minutes. Afterward, wash your face with a mild soap or cleanser. This treatment is not only good for your skin, but a great unwinder, too.

For tired eyes, another hazard of a nonstop schedule, try this soother. Apply cotton balls dipped in cooled chamomile tea to your closed lids. You may also want to steep washcloths in the remainder of the tea, then roll them up and store them in the refrigerator. When you need a refresher, pull one out and apply to your forehead or the back of your neck.

CHANGING YOUR ROUTINE

In addition to these suggested remedies for combatting stress, you can also give yourself a break by varying your usual work routine. After a taxing day, don't plunge right into the rush-hour traffic fight unless you absolutely have to. Window-shop, catch an early movie, or meet your husband or a friend for dinner. Or just stay at the office a little later to have some quiet time to unclutter your desk and do some reorganizing. That way you'll be more on top of things the next day.

If you have children to go home to, treat them to a quiet hour of play with you—reading stories or coloring pictures together—rather than diving into dinner preparations with them plucking at your sleeve. Order pizza or Chinese food so you won't have to cook, or pull some heat-and-serve stuff out of the freezer.

You can really unwind from the rigors of the office by involving yourself in a learning activity that demands a mental switch from what you do all day at work. Take a weaving course, learn to play a musical instrument, or join a political club. Whatever you choose, just make sure it is something you want to do, rather than something you feel you should do. "Should" tasks will make you feel further put-upon, while something you really want to get involved in will likely stimulate and recharge you.

Reserve weekends for the kind of rest and relaxation that allows you to push the pressures of the office aside. Use lunch hours and week-nights to run errands and take care of chores that would otherwise wipe out your weekend—things like laundry, grocery shopping, trips to the doctor and dentist, etc. Use waiting time or commuting time for little catch-up tasks, such as making lists of things to do or writing letters. And if you can, try to get away at least one weekend every month. You will be much better off for the change of pace and scenery.

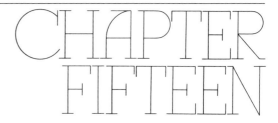

Finishing Your Day with TLC

The evening hours are a good time to attend to beauty upkeep. You would do well to establish a nighttime skin-care routine that includes both cleansing and moisturizing the face with products appropriate for your skin type. Nightly attention should also be given to special areas like the eyes and throat.

By shampooing and conditioning hair at night, you can add to your morning sleep time and not have to worry about drying your hair before you leave for the office. If your hair is damaged in any way, it will benefit from special treatments applied in the evening and left on while you sleep.

On a weekly rather than nightly basis, you might feel like pampering yourself with a complete manicure and/or pedicure. You can do either while watching TV or listening to music.

This chapter will outline how-tos for all of the above plus other grooming procedures, and also help you set up a routine for falling into a relaxed and peaceful sleep if you are usually the toss-and-turn type.

HAIR CARE

Clean hair is an essential aspect of the working woman's beauty image. Depending on your hair type and the condition it's in, that may mean shampooing every night. Contrary to what some people think, frequent shampooing is not damaging, provided you are careful to rinse your hair well.

To treat your hair right, choose a shampoo that is specially formulated for your hair type. Many shampoos come in four versions:

* Normal: to clean hair without drying it out
* Oily: to remove excess oil and condition hair without leaving it feeling greasy
* Dry or damaged: to provide the gentlest washing and the highest concentration of conditioners
* Antidandruff: containing zinc omadine or other flake-fighter ingredients

Choosing a shampoo with built-in conditioners saves the time and expense of an extra step.

When you shampoo, you should work suds into the scalp first, massaging vigorously with your fingertips (not nails). The reason a salon shampooing feels so good is because of the scalp massage that goes with it. Lots of lather isn't necessary, unless you're doing a TV commercial, nor is more than one washing. After lathering, run fingers through your hair to remove some tangles before rinsing. Use warm, not hot, water and rinse well. You don't need to get hair "squeaky clean"; if you do, it means your hair has been stripped of more than dirt. A final rinse with cool water will give hair more sheen.

Never use a brush on wet hair; it can cause breakage and split ends. Instead, use a wide-tooth comb and draw it through hair gently—no yanking. Towel off your hair and let it dry in the air for awhile before using a blow-dryer or electric rollers. This will prevent excessive dryness from too much heat on the hair. Remember to hold a blow-dryer at least 12 inches from the scalp, and adjust it to the cooler setting.

If your hair has a special problem, you may need to use a deep-penetrating conditioner once a month. Chemically treated hair should be conditioned every two to three weeks. There are many deep conditioners on the market for handling damaged hair, or you could try one of these simple home remedies:

MAYONNAISE TREATMENT. This is good for dry, coarse hair. You can make up a homemade mayonnaise with egg yolk, lemon juice, and oil or use the commercial product right out of the jar. Apply two or three tablespoons to the hair and comb through, then cover with a warm towel or plastic cap. Leave on at least 15 minutes, the longer the better. If your sleeping partner doesn't object, you can even keep it on overnight. Shampoo as usual after the treatment.

HOT OIL TREATMENT. This is good for all types of hair except very oily. You can use castor, mineral, or salad oil. One noted Manhattan hairdresser recommends baby oil with the contents of a capsule of vitamin E added. Heat the oil till it's warm to the touch, then part the hair in sections and apply to the entire scalp area. Cover your hair with a plastic cap or warm towel. Again, leave on as long as you can—a minimum of 10 minutes, overnight is great—then shampoo out.

UNWANTED HAIR

There are several do-it-yourself methods to deal routinely with unwanted hair, depending on its location on the body. Facial hair can be lightened with a cream bleach or whisked away with a brush-on hair remover. The brush feature facilitates a more uniform application of lotion for faster depilatory action.

Plucking stray brow hairs becomes less of a problem the more frequently you do it. Use a good mirror and a strong light, and pluck in the direction the hair grows. If brow area is sensitive, apply an ice cube for a few seconds or use a numbing gel like the kind rubbed on babies' gums during teething. Don't get carried away with plucking; you just want to remove stray hairs under the brow line and between the brows. Never pluck from above and always follow the line of your natural brow. Your aim is to clean up, not reshape.

For underarms and legs, you can use either a depilatory, electric shaver, or razor. Many razors are made specially for women with curved handles to give a smooth, nick-free shave on tricky spots like the kneecap. When you use a razor, make sure skin is wet and lubricated with soap or shaving cream. When using an electric shaver, skin should be free of all moisture. Don't borrow your husband's or roommate's razor. Not only is it unsanitary, but you may find dull blades, which can irritate skin. Use a razor with a clean, sharp blade, and shave against the direction of the hair growth, using long, even strokes. Go easy around ankles and shin bones, which are easily nicked. If you do cut yourself, just touch a styptic pencil to the nick to stop the bleeding. Don't put a piece of tissue over it; removing it may start the bleeding again.

After you shave your legs, be sure to apply a moisturizer to soothe and soften the skin. If you're doing a pedicure the same evening, it's nice to massage feet and legs together.

PEDICURE

A professional pedicure takes about an hour and costs around $15. But you can do an expert job yourself following these steps:

1. Take off any old polish. Use a gentle remover that doesn't strip nails of moisture.

2. Soak feet in warm, sudsy water. You can dangle them in the bathtub or use a small plastic basin. Use a pumice on heels, soles, and any other rough spots. Just make sure the pumice is wet or you'll rub off more than calluses. You might want to buy a battery-operated appliance with a whirring disk for smoothing.

3. Don't attempt to remove corns or treat ingrown toenails yourself. These are the province of a podiatrist. Also never pop a blister. Put a bandage over it until it opens itself.

4. While nails are still soft from soaking, clip them straight across. File rough edges in one direction with an emery board or battery appliance.

5. Never cut cuticles. It only encourages thicker regrowth. Instead, massage cuticle cream or remover all around the nail. Gently push back the cuticle with an orange stick wrapped in cotton. Use the stick to clean under nails, too.

6. Dunk feet in the water again, then pat them dry. Massage legs and feet with moisturizer following the technique outlined in the previous chapter. Pay special attention to the soles of the feet, where skin is likely to be toughest and need the most lubricating.

7. If you want to apply polish, wipe nails clean of moisturizer. Then twist and weave facial tissue or cotton balls between the toes to

separate them. Or invest a couple dollars in a pair of foam-rubber pads made with a groove for each toe. They're available at drug and department stores.

8. Apply base coat to give nails a smooth surface, follow with two coats of enamel. Bring polish right to the cuticle and clean up later with polish remover on a cotton-tipped stick. Finish with a clear top coat.

9. Relax with legs elevated until nails dry.

MANICURE

The procedure for a manicure is very similar to the one for the pedicure, but with a couple notable differences. To do a thorough job, follow these steps carefully, allowing about an hour if you plan to apply polish.

1. Again, start by removing old polish.

2. Holding an emery board at an angle so you're filing from underneath the tips of your nails, shape them into rounded ovals. File in one direction at a time, from the outside to the center—never back and forth or down at the corners of the nails. To prevent nails from splitting or peeling, keep them short, no more than a quarter of an inch beyond the fingertips, and all the same length. Nails should be filed when they are at their hardest, never after soaking in water. You don't want to cut or clip them, because the cells that make up nail plates are like stacks of paper and cutting results in ragged edges.

3. Massage cuticle cream thoroughly into the cuticles and the sides of the fingers. Soak nails for a few minutes in warm soapy water, then rinse and pat dry.

4. Dip a cotton-tipped swab or orange stick into cuticle remover and apply it around the cuticles and under the nails. Gently push back cuticles and clean under your nails. Leave scrubbing with nail brushes to surgeons; it weakens the nail surface.

5. Wash hands again to remove traces of cuticle remover. Trim hangnails with scissors. Don't cut cuticle if you can avoid it, because it will grow out ragged and cause more hangnails.

6. If you're using polish, brush on a clear base coat, doing the thumb first, little finger next, and then working back to the other three. Cover the entire nail with a light coat and let it dry until it is slick to the touch.

7. Apply polish in the same sequence of fingers as you did the base. Use three light strokes: one down the center of each nail, then one down each side. Let the first coat dry for a few minutes, then apply another. Wait until the second coat is fairly dry before attempting to clean up any overrun with a cotton swab dipped in polish remover.

8. Finish with a clear top coat or sealer, bringing it up, over, and under the edge of the nail. Give polish a chance to dry before doing anything with your hands or going to bed; otherwise you're likely to mar the surface.

When polish is properly applied and given plenty of time to dry, a manicure should last a week to 10 days. Though the surface dries in a few minutes, it takes some 12 hours for polish to harden clear through.

Doing a manicure before bedtime is a good idea because it gives polish a chance to set during the night. For most working situations, a transparent nail tint is probably more acceptable than dark-colored enamel. Also chips won't be so noticeable if you're not able to repair them immediately.

The use of polish can actually strengthen nails, particularly if you choose a formula with built-in conditioners. Polish serves as a protection to the nails and can help seal splits together. But don't leave polish on too long or add fresh coats over old. Always start with clean nails. Also, don't pick at polish. Since nails grow in layers, picking can peel off the top layer.

Be sure you wipe the neck of the bottle each time you use it and twist the cap back on firmly. Polish that has thickened in the bottle can be restored by adding a few drops of enamel solvent. Don't use polish remover for this purpose.

SKIN CARE

Your nightly skin-care routine should consist of three steps: cleansing, toning, and moisturizing. For **oily skin**, wash face with a mild cleansing bar or a lotion cleanser that can be rinsed off with water. Then wipe on astringent with a cotton pad to remove excess oil from the surface of your skin. Pay special attention to the problem areas of your face: nose, chin, and forehead. Even oily skin gets thirsty for moisture. Choose a lightweight emulsion that slips quickly into the skin, leaving it feeling supple and velvety.

Partly dry, partly oily skin should also be washed with a cleansing bar or rinse-off lotion cleanser. Saturate a cotton pad with astringent and wipe it over nose, chin, and forehead. Use a toner for your cheeks; it's invigorating but doesn't strip moisture from the dry skin there. Finally, choose a lightweight emulsion to soothe and soften your skin. A heavy lubricant is the last thing you want to put on your face.

Normal to slightly dry skin needs a creamy cleanser to dissolve makeup. Use this soothing, lightweight lotion to remove makeup gently without harmful scrubbing. Massage all over face and throat, then tissue or rinse off. If you don't have much makeup to remove, you can wash your face with a gentle cleansing bar. Use a toner to wipe away the last traces of cleanser and prepare skin for its moisture treatment. Saturate a cotton pad and run it over the area you've just cleansed. Then saturate a second pad and pat it lightly but purposefully on face and throat. To replace vital moisture while you sleep, finish with a lightweight cream or moisturizing emulsion.

Dry to very dry skin types should use a creamy cleanser or very gentle soap as described in the preceding paragraph. Follow cleansing by smoothing an alcohol-free freshener over face and throat with a cotton pad. Choose a formula with only the mildest ingredients and skin-soothing emollients. About 20 minutes before bedtime, apply night cream all over your face, using upward motions. This is a must for very dry skin. At times when your skin is not so dry, you can use a lightweight cream instead.

In addition to regular cleansing, oily and combination skin will profit from an application of an astringent facial mask two or three times a week (more often if skin is very oily). A mask like this will control excess oil, unclog and refine pores. Skin in the normal to dry or very dry range can enjoy the benefits of a creamy clay facial mask. Used once a week, this kind of mask will slough off dry, dead surface cells and leave a finer finish to the skin. It tones, tightens, and brightens without drying.

If you're doing an at-home facial routine, a mask is a good follow-up to a steam treatment. Fill a basin with hot water and lean over it for a few minutes with a towel over your head like a tent. This helps open pores and prepares your face to receive the full benefits of the mask. You can also buy facial saunas to steam the skin, as well as brushes and battery-operated appliances with various attachments to aid in cleaning and massaging your face.

There are certain skin-care needs that cross all skin-type boundaries. The most acute is the care of the eye area. This part of the face lacks natural oil glands and fat underneath the surface. It yearns constantly for moisture.

Since the skin around the eyes is some of the most delicate on the body, it makes good sense to handle it with care. Never pull or rub. Use special eye makeup remover to wipe away mascara and all traces of shadow and liner. Stroke it on lightly with your finger, then smooth a bit more down over your lashes. Use a soft cloth or cotton and the same kind of strokes to wipe it away. Then lubricate the area by tapping on an eye wrinkle cream in a circular pattern. Or use your eye oil wrinkle stick. Finish by using an emollient lash cream as a lubricant/moisturizer/protein treatment for dry, brittle lashes. Helena Rubinstein's version is packaged in an automatic mascara-type dispenser.

The neck and throat are another area deficient in oil glands and potentially rich in wrinkles. That's why it is never too early to get into a nightly routine of massaging neck cream into the skin. Begin at the base of the throat and work up to the chin line with long, languid strokes.

For the last step in your every-night routine, slather on some hand cream. Choose a nongreasy formula that is quickly absorbed.

TEETH

Proper brushing and flossing of your teeth is also essential. Most dentists recommend using a soft-bristle brush with a flat brushing surface. For flossing, mentally divide your mouth into four sections. Floss half of the upper teeth from front to back of the mouth, then do the other half. Repeat with the lower teeth. The first few times you try flossing, you may find it a little awkward and your gums may bleed and be sore. But this is only a temporary condition. If bleeding should continue, consult your dentist; you may be doing something wrong.

Besides this at-home routine, you should see a dentist twice a year to have teeth cleaned and plaque—the substance that builds up on the teeth—removed. If you don't, you are risking periodontal disease, the greatest cause of tooth loss in adults. Researchers estimate that 20 percent of all young adults and more than 90 percent of the middle-aged population in this country suffers from some form of this disease. Since it is rarely painful in its early stages, many people don't realize they are harboring the disease until it's too late and expensive and painful treatments are necessary. The best insurance for your teeth is to practice preventive measures now.

SLEEP

Insomnia affects virtually all of us some of the time, and about 25 million Americans all of the time. If you are someone who lies in bed without falling asleep or wakes up during the night and can't drop back off, you are likely to find your days disrupted as well as your nights. When you sleep poorly, you probably feel dragged out and unable to function at your best level the following day.

Many people with this problem reach for sleeping pills (insomniacs support a $100 million-a-year industry in this country) or down a couple drinks, hoping this will help them nod off. Unfortunately, neither of these "treatments" is a long-term solution. In fact, they can have adverse effects on your sleep patterns, actually making insomnia worse.

Instead, start by changing any poor bedtime habits that you might have. Try to go to bed at the same time each night. Studies show that keeping regular hours helps you drop off more quickly and sleep more soundly. Don't drink too much coffee or other beverages containing caffeine, like tea or colas, late in the day. Coffee lovers should try to switch to a decaffeinated brand, while tea drinkers can investigate herbal teas available in health-food stores and many supermarkets. Chamomile and spearmint teas are said to have a soporific effect, and drinking a cup of either before bedtime can be a soothing habit to get into. You might also try drinking a glass of milk, preferably warm. Milk contains "tryptophan," a substance which promotes sleep. It will help if you don't eat a big meal, exercise vigorously, or discuss disturbing topics shortly before retiring. If you've brought work home from the office, knock off at least a half hour before bedtime to give your mind a chance to gear down.

Normally, people fall asleep within 10 to 15 minutes of going to bed. If you find yourself still awake after an hour, it may be because you're too tense. Try this relaxation exercise:

Close your eyes and focus your attention on your right arm. Say to yourself, "My arm feels warm and heavy." Try to feel the warmth spreading up your arm from your fingertips to your shoulders. Try this with the other arm, saying the same words, then move on to other parts of the body—your head, shoulders, stomach, legs, feet. If this doesn't work for you, try another variation. Start by tensing your right arm, with your hand in a fist. Make it very tight and hold for a few seconds, then release. Repeat the tense-relax pattern with other body parts.

When you're trying to relax, let your mind help your body. Block out irrelevant thoughts and concentrate on your muscles and relaxing them. If you can't keep your mind from wandering, let it flow to a tranquil scene. Imagine every detail of it: water lapping against rocks, a field of wheat waving in the breeze, a blue sky full of billowing white clouds.

If you still can't sleep, you might as well get up for awhile rather than toss and turn. Smooth out the sheets and blankets and go into another room to read or do something else. If you have been unable to stop thinking about a particular problem, try writing down possible solutions or courses of action you can take. This may relieve your anxieties enough to permit sleep.

Don't worry too much about missed sleep when it only happens occasionally. Each of us has a strong reserve of sleep, just as we have a food reserve. You don't die of starvation if you fast for a few days, nor will you suffer any dire consequences if you don't get your customary 40 winks every night.

Different people have different sleep needs, and we supposedly require less as we get older. If you suddenly find yourself waking up an hour earlier than usual day after day, it may be because your requirements have readjusted. Instead of worrying about it, be grateful you have an extra hour in which to get things done.

Experiments at Tufts University point to different personality traits between long and short sleepers. Boredom is believed to drive some people to sleep for extended periods, while it is possible for us to get by with less sleep, provided our lives interest us. Those who need eight hours or more tend to be critical, complain of minor aches and pains, and be worriers. Conversely, those who can get by on six hours or less were found to be efficient and ambitious. They work hard, are self-assured, sociable, and satisfied with their lives.

In the end, it seems that having a job you like and are involved with, and being eager to face each new day put you in a state of mind more invigorating even than sleep. And maybe that's the working woman's biggest beauty bonus of all.